LEAN AND GREEN DIET COOKBOOK

Transform Your Health, Lose Weight Fast and Turn Your Body into a Fat-Burning Machine with a Selection of Delicious, Simple and Wholesome Recipes

28-Day Meal Plan Included

By **Healthy Food Lab.**

Table of Content

INTRODUCTION

Many people would love to wave a magic wand and be able to take care of their meals for the rest of their life. On Medi-fast, 5 of your six meals are made and prepared for you, so this diet does not entail much cooking, shopping, or planning, and is very simple and effective.

You are still responsible for your lean and green meal. This is the one fresh meal you make each day or every other day, not counting a frozen meal or going out to a restaurant. Some people would prefer not to have this meal cooked, but substitute a large salad or smoothie instead.

You're probably wondering if the Medi-fast diet can be practiced during meals or at restaurants. This is possible and the secret to this is to truly understand the food and nutrition requirements. One of the simplest times to eat Medi-fast is when you usually eat your "lean and green meal" during the day.

Crash or fad diets are still used today, even though they are highly ineffective in the long term. While crash diets work for a little while, failure to do them properly can cause more harm than good in the long term.

CHAPTER ONE

The Green Diet

There is a wide variety of foods that can reduce the risk of inflammation and help weight-controlling hormones function to the best of their ability, which in turn regulates our appetite and manages our blood sugar. These types of foods include, but are not limited to, berries, vegetables, fatty fish, nutrients, seeds, as well as their oils, whole grains, and spices.

- Herbs and spices are valuable because they are rich in antioxidants, which protect cells from the damage inflicted when inflammatory cells are attacking the body. Antioxidants form a shield around our body's cells and absorb free radicals, which lose their destructive energy and are securely excreted from the body.

- You can see free radical harm happening if you split an apple in half and leave one half uncovered for 20 minutes. The apple begins to get brown and dries as it reacts with the oxygen in the air, which produces free radicals. However, it preserves its white color and texture if you soak the other half in lemon juice. This is because it is covered in vitamin C which is an excellent antioxidant.

- The antioxidant-rich, anti-inflammatory properties of spices and herbs promote fat burning while fat accumulation is reduced. They also add taste and excitement to food and reduce the intake of salt. Too much salt contributes to fluid accumulation, another adversary to fat loss.

- For every diet we start, there are so many new items on the shopping list to find. A simple way to start with new ingredients for the Medi-fast diet is buying frozen fruits and vegetables. Frozen fruits and vegetables are filled with just as much nutrient punch as their fresh counterparts. You can make soups and smoothies really easily if you have a few bags available in your freezer! If we already have at least six bags of frozen fruit and vegetables in the freezer, we've got a good head start on planning healthy meals. Not all of your fruits and veggies need to be frozen, but by having frozen food on hand, you always have a backup plan for your meals.

-When hunger strikes, we drink frozen green tea paired with fresh fruit juice and sparkling water. Why it works: Hunger and thirst are sometimes confused. A glass of water can stave our hunger, but it's nice to broaden our horizons with the types of beverages we drink. Caffeine-rich green tea combined with sweet, fresh juice rich in vitamins and fizzy water is a new and exciting concept.

-Having snacks on hand is helpful, and just having an apple and a bag of almonds can make a difference in your day. Apples (and pears) are high in pectin, leading to fat absorption; they are also abundant insoluble fibers, which slow down sugar absorption into the bloodstream. Almonds are a perfect mix of protein/essential fat. The two together make a healthy, fat-burning, and filling snack.

What Is A Lean and Green Diet?

What is a green and lean meal?
A Lean & Green meal consists of 5 to 7 ounces of cooked lean protein plus three portions of non-starchy vegetables and up to two portions of healthy fats, depending on your preference for lean protein. Enjoy the Lean & Green meal every day and choose anything that fits best for your schedule. A lean and green meal consists of 5 to 7 ounces of cooked lean protein plus three portions of non-starchy and up to two portions of healthy fats, depending on your preference for lean protein. You will enjoy your lean & green meal(s), which best fit your schedule, for each of your six meals during the day.

Healthy Fats
Add up to two portions of healthy fats to your Lean & Green meal every day. Healthy fat is important because it maintains the body's fat stores, but in a more balanced way. Through healthy fat, the body absorbs A, D, E, and K vitamins. These vitamins help the bladder function properly.

People want to know if they should miss this meal or replace one of the prepackaged "Medi-fast meals" with the lean and the green meal. People have often questioned if they should only use a frozen meal to fulfill this requirement since they want their food to be cooked for them. In the following post, I will answer these concerns.

Why do people think of missing or replacing Lean and Green Food? I have several explanations, but the most common ones are here. Often, people believe they save calories or carbohydrates when they introduce a sixth meal. Or, people often really get used to not having to cook their own food, and they find that they enjoy it. Getting their work completed allows them not to stress about food or think about it. Basically, they go into a groove where the diet really clicks and works for them, and they won't disturb it by having to eat a bigger meal.

I appreciate these two issues only as I myself had them. But here, I did not understand that the five pre-packed foods you consume the rest of the day are so low in calories (100 per 500 per day in total) that when you eat the main meal, you have plenty of room for extra calories. There is plenty of space to be flexible with a good amount of protein (5 to 7 ounces) and some vegetables. You don't have to skimp. You can still eat fresh food and take in a minimal amount of calories.

I also get people who want to use a frozen meal, such as Lean Cuisine or some other brand, to fulfill the requirement. This is not the right idea, the organization says, and I have to agree. It's all about having fresh food. One way to succeed in this is to learn how to make healthier decisions and how to plan nutritious meals. You will eventually have to learn this ability anyway and it is better to start now.

The lean and green meal does not have to be either hard or inconvenient. You can make it very easily by cooking a little lean meat and salad on the side. Or you can get elaborate and benefit from many recipes. There is a lot of flexibility here but knowing what the requirements are is crucial. The organization wants you to eat nutritious food, with fresh ingredients, and they want you to learn how to cook it so that you hold the weight off in the long term.

Are Premade Lean and Green Meals Available?
Some people don't want to cook a lean and green meal once a day. I am often asked if Medi-fast offers ready-made or frozen lean and green meals. The business does not sell ready-made products that can be used as a full meal as of right now. The goal of the program is to lose your target weight and leave the plan, this would become difficult if you were solely relying on Medi-fast to provide your meals.

In order to maintain your weight loss goals you would need to know how to schedule and prepare balanced meals. Responsibility for a nutritious meal every day is a simple way to do so. But this doesn't mean that you will have to labor in the kitchen every day.

The lean and green meal requirement doesn't have to be difficult or complicated. If you note that the meal is just lean protein and three low carbohydrate vegetables, it's a little simpler. You can use food from a restaurant or frozen food if you have carefully picked them. You don't want frozen food or foods full of carbon dioxide, preservatives, sodium, and fat in your restaurant. You might have to read labels and analyze your choices, in a very realistic way. You can also buy pre-packaged food from the grocery store. Try a cut of lean roast meat with a basic bagged salad, it takes just a couple of minutes, and that's all you need. Pre-packaged meals are also simple, but be sure to check the ingredients so that you are getting the best quality possible. Easy soups and stews are also a good simple meal, as long as you use lean meat, beans and lots of vegetables.

As a result, Medi-fast has no ready or frozen lean and green foods to answer the question asked, but they can easily be prepared using pre-packaged foods from the grocery store or frozen or restaurant foods. As you transition from the diet, learning to select your own fresh foods would really help you.

How to Get Lean Diet Tips
4 Tips to Help You Get Super Lean, Fast!

This section will help you accomplish your goals if you are searching for easy ways to get lean. If you follow these diet guidelines, you must be consistent and diligent, but the results will be more than worthwhile.

Lean Diet Tips #1: How to Get Lean
Priority protein – Protein is valuable to protect muscle mass. The more muscle you get, the more calories you are going to burn. Concentrate on having at least 1 gram of protein per pound of your current body weight. Nutrition holds you longer, too. For these tough hungry times, a meal is supplemented by a low-carbon protein drink.

Tips #2: How to Get Lean Diet

Low glycemic and low-calorie vegetables offer you slow-burning energy. Vegetables are an essential aspect of weight-loss and a great way to avoid snacking on unhealthy foods.

Tips # 3: How to Get Lean Diet

Lose weight with water - Yes, the process of weight loss can be improved with plenty of water. It extracts fat from the cells and removes unnecessary contaminants from the bodies. 8 - 12 glasses a day is a good guide to follow every day. Water is also going to suppress your appetite and discourage you from eating.

How to Get Lean Diet Tips # 4:

Include healthy fats, this is vital because some people are afraid to eat fats. There are different types of healthy fats which occur naturally in many different types of natural foods. Try to consume 5-7 grams of fat per meal.

It's easy to lose weight quickly when you know how.

CHAPTER TWO
Diet for Women to Get Lean

Why Are You Still Struggling to Get Toned?

What if you could have a diet that helps to get your muscle toned and energized? Did you know that diets are mostly to help us find a functional meal plan to help us maintain our weight? Many people think dieting is about looking a certain way, and it's unfortunate that a lot of people work hard in the gym but can't lower their body fat. Due to their poor eating habits, no matter how much they work out, they can't seem to lose the weight.

Did you know you could lose muscle mass if you did not eat enough protein? Nutrition is often overlooked when trying to get in shape. Protein is a necessary form of food to get lean.

If there is insufficient protein will it cause you to store fat? Are you getting enough protein to lose fat in your diet?

Nutrition, carbs, and fats in their proper proportions are important for getting in shape. However, the amount of protein is particularly important. You need so much more than carbohydrates and fats. One of the first criteria of your lean muscle diet is to improve your consumption of protein. All of your body – skin, hair, muscle, etc. consists of protein.

By slowly building muscle, you can work toward the lean and toned body you aspire to achieve. The amount of muscle that you have influences your metabolism directly. Through eating protein, regularly working out and incorporating weight lifting into your exercise routine, you can gradually add muscle to your body.

It is a commonly known fact that working with weights builds muscle quickly. When you lift weights or work out, your muscle tissue breaks down. The body will then heal, restore and recover the muscles.

Your body takes the protein you eat in your diet and splits it into amino acids so that your muscles can rebuild them wherever necessary. This is what makes the muscles sculpted and visible. This is a natural process, but only if you have enough protein in your diet. If you don't have enough protein, your body breaks down your existing muscle to refuel from your workout.

A healthy diet should not neglect protein intake. This may be the missing link if you don't see a rise in muscle mass. Do you go to the gym religiously but don't see the results you want? It might be time to review your protein intake.

In general, the best diet is around 50-60 grams of protein per day. This can also be expressed in 0.8 grams of protein per kilogram of body weight. If you build your body as you are, your body weight is 0.85 pounds.

Diet to Get Lean for Women
You May Not Be Eating Enough to Lose Weight

Are you eating enough to build healthy muscle mass? Did you know you can keep your body from losing weight if you don't eat enough? This is a common misunderstanding. Many people assume that they can lose weight by not eating. This is not always true, however. Let us see if this misunderstanding has been corrected.

Some common questions that come up are, "shouldn't I eat less to lose weight?" or "how do I eat more often and continue to lose weight?"

Surprisingly, it is best to eat a small meal or snack every three to four hours if you are trying to lose weight.

When you wait for more than four hours and then eat, the next meal you eat will be stored in your body, whether high or low in nutrition. When you consume nutritious meals (high protein, lower carbohydrates, and fats), the metabolism accelerates into a combustion mode every 4 hours.

A good way to look at it is that however much you eat (you can think of the food as "fueling" your body) your body is more likely to keep extra fat burning, especially if the food is nutritious and easy to digest. The loss in muscle mass thus leads to a slower metabolism. The more wood (fuel) in a fire, the more fire you burn. Remove wood, and the fire is going to go out!

Muscle is the only place you burn calories in your body. As muscle mass is increased by eating and exercising, metabolism is also increase. You can burn calories even in a state of inactivity. When your body is hungry or fasting (no food for more than 4 hours), it preserves food that has been converted into energy into body fat for emergencies.

Another downside to hunger is that your body takes its supply of energy from the essential tissue, such as your brain, skin, muscle, and inner organ mass. Therefore, your best diet to get lean should include adequate protein, particularly after training, to repair and reconstruct your muscles. Bear in mind, however, that if not eating often enough you will experience:

The body being in a state of deprivation

Reducing fat-burning metabolism and decreasing muscle mass when expending energy

Sacrifice of organ tissue energy

Depriving your body of protein, which is essential for repair and reconstruction of muscle mass

In order to keep up with these dietary needs, increase protein intake by including basic protein shakes into your meal plan. This increases your stamina, helps you to sleep better, and avoids all the above issues if you tend to skip meals or snacks.

Protein shakes are a simple and convenient way to stabilize your nutrient and protein intake throughout the day.

Carry a few scoops of protein powder with you while you're on the go. Add water, juice, or milk.

Protein stabilizes the blood sugar level all day long.

Protein raises the metabolism rate - maintains weight loss and muscle build-up

Protein shakes prevent you from snacking unhealthily

Protein drinks provide the required nutrients and energy without consuming a meal

What If I Don't Have Time to Make the Lean and Green Meal?

Often these questions include a type of deception, when people would rather avoid the meal than make it. I heard a short time ago from someone who said: "I am an accountant, and during the fiscal time I have to skip a lot of dinners."

There are so many excuses that people give to skip out on making their own lean and green meal, but the truth is, it's easier to learn how to make it now in order to sustain your weight loss in the long term.

What if you're not making excuses but just skipping your lean and green because you're working and you can't fit the time in to cook for yourself? Don't be too hard on yourself if you can't make it. Just do the best you can, and try to carry on in the morning.

Can You Have Vegetarian Lean and Green Meals on ?

Often, I hear from people who consider Medi-fast's diet, who are either vegetarians or who are trying to reduce the amount of meat that they consume. One common question is whether you can make a vegetarian lean and green meal, or whether meat is required to make it?

This diet is ideal for catering to vegetarians. You absolutely don't need to have any meat or animal products in your lean and green meal. They have clear documentation for vegetarians on how to make a lean green meal work.

The company recommends using veggie burgers, veggie sausage, and veggie chicken patties in place of meat. Using the proposed amount of portion size and three portions of vegetables, everything you might use as vegetarian protein will work.

All of Medi-fast's prepackaged foods, such as shakes, puddings, oatmeal's, bars, and snacks are vegetarian to start with. This makes it quite simple to be on the Medi-fast diet as a vegetarian and you don't have to have meat with your lean and green meal. The diet is structured to be very versatile. Essentially, you need just three rations of low glycemic vegetables and one portion of protein, whether vegetarian or otherwise.

What is the Lean and Green Meal?

This is part of keeping your calories in balance, but also inconsistently feeding, in order to maintain your metabolism as high as it can be. Many people in the diet use the 5 plus 1 diet, which means five meals and a bigger lean and green meal. Two lean and green meals would go against the five-plus one plan, but there is enough flexibility within the diet that you can accommodate it to your needs. All of this is to produce the best results when setting things up so that you can thrive on your diet and live a healthy lifestyle.

In order to do this, you want a happy medium to be established. The 5 plus 1 plan is prepared so that about 550 to 550 calories are served with five dietary foods; the remaining calories are lean and green, containing 5-7 ounces of protein and three vegetables. If you still want to be on the five-plus 1, you might divide it into two pieces. Or, you might just know that you are making a hybrid plan, and you realize that even with two slender and green ones, you probably still take a lot fewer calories and carbs and get the corresponding results.

Finally, there is a meal plan for Medi-fast, which reflects this dilemma. The 4 plus 2 is named, and there are 4 Medi-fast prepackaged meals and two meals of lean and green. Nevertheless, I have to be frank and tell you that the four-plus two are mostly used by people who have been on a diet for some time, lost the weight they had hoped to lose, and now move from the diet. But again, nobody will ask you to justify yourself. If you have two bigger meals, check to see what kind of results you receive. You just want to make sure you eat lean, green foods and lean protein, and low glycemic vegetables carefully. And, if you have the chance, promise to do as well as possible. This young woman, for example, will not eat with customers every day of the week. She could try the five-plus one process on her days off if she wanted it.

But it was very likely that the four-plus two would fit well for her. Many people are pleased with the 4 plus 2 findings. And even with two lean and green meals, this typically only means slightly less calories and carbohydrates for most people. This results in loss of weight without too much sacrifice or a shift in lifestyle.

One of the first questions anyone contemplating the Medi-fast diet is: 'What is the green & lean meal?' This is the only meal that you cook per day and consume it in addition to five servings of Medi-fast meals a day.

Medi-fast is planned in a way that substitutes a low-fat meal with a minimal calorie. They name their daily 5 and 1 plans since it includes the five meal substitutes per day and one meal, which you make of lean protein, fresh greens, and vegetables.

Lean and green food is your opportunity to start experimenting with healthy food options and how to manage portion sizes. It also means that you get to try a new meal every day, which is an integral part of the Medi-fast schedule. If you plan your lean & green menu for the week, you can have lunch and dinner without worrying about slipping on your schedule.

Each lean and green contains a portion of lean protein and a portion of fresh greens and vegetables. Medi-fast likes to explain this by saying that you cut a plate in half and fill the protein on one side and the vegetables on the other. However, our focus is also on portion control here, depending on what kind of protein and vegetables you plan to eat.

Depending on your selection, the protein part is anywhere from 5 to 7 ounces on the lean side of your meal. For example, you would have a 5-ounce portion if you wanted to get lean beef or pork chop. You will have a portion of six ounces for skinless chicken breast, tofu, or swordfish, and you would also have a portion of fat, like a teaspoon of olive oil and two tablespoons in a low-carb dressing.

You can have 7 ounces of food in protein that are very light in fat, such as the different white fishes (Cod, Haddock, Tilapia, etc.), shellfish, and gamma meats like buffalo plus two fat serving portions. You can broil your fish with olive oil, and then you can dress up in a nice big salad on the side.

Now to the green side of the board. You are recommended to have three servings of greens a day, all at one meal! One serving is one cup of raw vegetables, which counts lettuce, spinach, collards, and all other salad greens. Servings are 1/2 cup for other vegetables, either raw or cooked.

If you want a half-nice salad, two cups of greens such as Romanesque and spinach can be put together. Add a half-cup of raw vegetables, such as onions, peas, and radishes. Don't like salad? Try 1/2 cup of sliced mushrooms and one cup of fresh asparagus sauteed in olive oil and lemon!

CHAPTER THREE:
LEAN AND GREEN DIET RECIPES

Breakfast Recipes

Tomato Kale and Egg Muffin

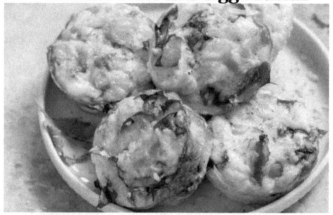

Ready in: 35 mins

Yield: 4 Servings

Per Serving: 1 Leaner, 1 Healthy Fat, 3 Green & 1 Condiment

Ingredients

8 eggs

3/4 cup low-fat Greek yogurt

1 cup egg whites

1/3 teaspoon salt

1 1/2 cups chopped roma tomatoes

1 (10-oz) package frozen chopped kale, thawed and patted dry

2 oz feta cheese, crumbled

Instructions

Preheat your oven to 375 F.

Combine the egg whites, yogurt, cheese, and salt in a bowl.

Add in the kale and chopped tomatoes

Lightly spray 20-cup muffin tin and pour the mixture into each well.

Bake the muffin for about 25 minutes or until s toothpick inserted in the center comes out clean.

Serve. Enjoy!

Nutritional Facts per Serving

289 calories; 14.8g fat; 10.9g fat; 29g protein.

Broccoli Almond Breakfast Bake

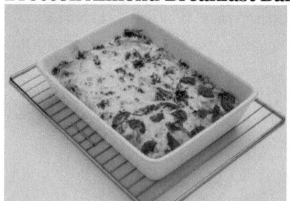

Ready in: 55 mins

Yield: 4 Servings

1 Lean, 3 Green, 1.5 Condiments

Ingredients

8 eggs

2 1/2 tablespoons of water

2 medium heads broccoli, cut into florets

3/4 cup unsweetened almond milk

Salt and ground black pepper to taste

1 cup part-skim/low-fat mozzarella, shredded

1/4 teaspoon cayenne pepper

Instructions

Preheat your oven to 375 F.

Place the broccoli florets in a microwave-safe bowl. Add in 2 1/2 tablespoons of water and microwave on high for about 4 minutes until tender.

Transfer the cooked broccoli to a colander to drain off any excess liquid.

While the broccoli is cooking, combine the eggs, almond milk, cayenne, salt, and ground pepper in a bowl.

Place the broccoli in a lightly greased baking dish. Sprinkle over the Mozzarella, and then pour the egg mixture on top.

Bake in the preheated oven for at least 40 minutes or until set in the middle and brown at the top.

Nutritional Facts per Serving

291 calories; 8.3g carbs; 24.6g protein; 18g fat.

Peppermint Mocha Shake

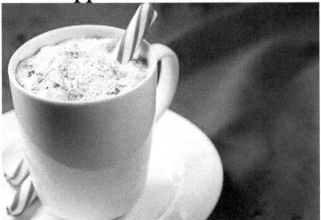

Ready in: 5 mins

Yield: 1 Serving

1 Fueling, 1.5 condiments

Ingredients

1 sachet Optavia Essential Creamy Chocolate Shake

1/4 cup unsweetened almond milk

1/2 teaspoon peppermint syrup

1 cup brewed coffee

1/4 teaspoon cinnamon

1 1/2 tablespoons low-fat whipped cream.

Instructions

Mix the chocolate, coffee, and almond in a small bowl.

Stir very well until the chocolate is completely dissolved.

Add in the peppermint and stir.

Serve in a mug topped with whipped cream and a sprinkle of cinnamon.

Nutritional Facts

87 calories; 5.4g fat; 4g protein; 4g carbs.

White Chicken Chili

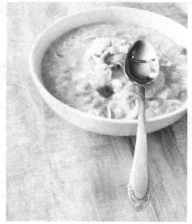

PREP TIME 15 mins

COOK TIME 45 mins

TOTAL TIME an hr

Ingredients

1 16 oz can great northern beans (drained)

2 lbs cooked, chopped chicken

2 yellow onions (chopped)

5 cloves garlic (minced)

3 cups chicken broth

1 can green chilies (drained)

2 tsp chili powder

1/3 cup chopped jalapenos (no seeds)

1 tbsp cumin

1 tbsp cayenne pepper

1 tbsp Worcestershire sauce

1 tbsp Tabasco

2 tsp oregano

1 16oz can chopped tomatoes (drained)

salt and pepper to taste

Directions

White Chicken Chili Sauté Onion and garlic until clear.

Cook. Add other ingredients and cook over medium heat.

Remove every 10 minutes until mixture is well blended and mixed (about 45 minutes)

Add If your white chili is too thick, add additional chicken broth.

Nutrition

Carbohydrates: 89.5 g

Calories: 557.0 kcal

Saturated Fat: 3.4 g

Protein: 44.2 g

Serving Unit: bowl

Serving Amount: 1

Sodium: 271.0 mg

Green Hummus

Prep Time: 15 minutes

Cook Time: 0 minutes

Yield: 1 1/2 cups (12 ounces)

INGREDIENTS

For the green hummus*

1 15-ounce can chickpeas (or 1 1/2 cups cooked)

1 small garlic clove

2 green onions

1/4 cup lime juice (2 limes)

2 cups baby spinach leaves

1/2 cup packed cilantro leaves and tender stems

1/4 teaspoon cumin

1/4 cup tahini

1/4 cup aquafaba (can liquid from the chickpeas), plus more as needed

3/4 teaspoon kosher salt

For the garnish

Crispy Chickpeas, cilantro leaves, Olive oil

Directions

1. Skin the garlic, drain the chickpeas into a cup of fluid calculation. Juice the limes. Cut the green onions, including the greens, into 1-inch bits.

2. In a food processor, add the garlic, cilantro, green onion, and spinach until finely chopped. Stir in the lime juice, chickpeas, cumin, tahini, kosher salt, and chickpea broth (aquafaba). Then scrape the bowl down for 30 seconds. Good taste. Add 1 to 2 tablespoons aquafaba if necessary. Puree to a smooth consistency for 1 to 2 minutes. Store cool for 7 to 10 days.

3. Top hummus, as needed, with cilantro leaves, olive oil drizzle, and crispy chickpeas. Serve with pita bread, veggies, and crackers

BEST Glowing Green Smoothie

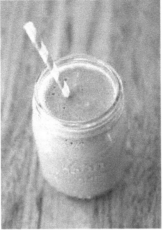

Prep Time: 5 minutes

Cook Time: 0 minutes

Yield: 2 cups (1 large or 2 small smoothies)

Ingredients

1 tablespoon maple syrup

1 large green apple

1/4 cup raw cashews

1/2 cup water

10 ice cubes

3 cups spinach

1 tablespoon fresh squeezed lemon juice

Directions

1. Cut the apple into pieces and leave the skin on.

2. Combine and blend all ingredients. Apply the lemon juice and mix again for a few seconds. Taste add a drop of maple syrup and/or lemon juice if you wish. Serve immediately or cool until one day.

Vibrant Spring Soup

Prep Time: 10 minutes

Cook Time: 30 minutes

Yield: 4 to 6

Ingredients

1 teaspoon ground cumin

1 tablespoon olive oil

1 large yellow onion, chopped

1 teaspoon ground coriander

3 garlic cloves, minced

Kosher salt

10 small new potatoes, cut into small cubes

2 ribs celery, thinly sliced

Juice of 1/2 lemon

Freshly ground black pepper

1 pound fresh or frozen English peas

4 cups vegetable broth

2 to 3 green onions or chives, thinly sliced, for garnish

4 cups baby spinach

Handful mint leaves, chopped (optional)

Directions

1. Heat the oil over the medium heat in a medium soup pot. Add the cumin, coriander, onion, and a few pins of salt.

2. Toast the garlic, celery, potatoes, salt, and black pepper and cook, stirring, until fragrant for another five minutes. Add the citrus juice and allow it to absorb for 1 minute, and then pour into the vegetable broth or water.

3. Bring the stock to a boil, cook the heat to a cooler, and cover the potatoes for 10 to 15 minutes until it is tender. Apply to the soup the peas and greens and blend until the greens go down.

4. Transfer to the blender 1 1/2 cup of soup and mix until smooth. Return the mixed soup to the pot and mix. Taste seasonings and change them if necessary. Serve the soup with cabbage, fresh mint, and a lemon squeeze.

Zesty Green Goddess Dressing

Prep Time: 5 minutes

Cook Time: 0 minutes

Yield: About 1 cup

Ingredients

½ green jalapeño pepper

2 green onions (scallions)

½ cup lightly packed cilantro

⅔ cup Greek yogurt

⅓ cup olive oil

Juice from 1 lime (2 tablespoons)

1 tablespoon maple syrup or honey

½ teaspoon kosher salt

Directions

1.Chop the green onions. Seed the jalapeño pepper and dice it.

2. In the cup of an immersion blender, put the green onions and jalapeno pepper in the (or in a blender). Add Greek yogurt, coriander, lime juice, kosher salt, olive oil, and maple syrup or honey. Blend to blend. Shift to an airtight container; store the dressing for one week in the refrigerator.

Green Pea Dip (Party Favorite!)

Prep Time: 5 minutes

Cook Time: 0 minutes

Yield: 2 1/2 cups

Ingredients

1 large bunch cilantro (about 3 cups packed leaves and stems)

1 pound frozen peas

3/4 teaspoon kosher salt

1 cup mild salsa verde

For dipping: pita chips, Tortilla chips, homemade crostini, or crackers

Directions

1. thaw the peas.

2. In a food processor, mix all ingredients and process to blend; scrape the bowl and process until smooth again. When appropriate, taste and change the flavors, adding extra cilantro and salsa to your liking. Up to 3 days of refrigerated storage.

Roasted Tomatillo Salsa (Salsa Verde)

Prep Time: 10 minutes

Cook Time: 10 minutes

Yield: 1 cup

Ingredients

1/2 serrano chile (or more, to taste)

8 ounces tomatillos

Handful fresh cilantro

2 large garlic cloves

1/2 teaspoon kosher salt

1 small white onion

Directions

1. Remove the tomatillos from the paper and rinse them. From the serrano chile, cut the stem. Peel the cloves of garlic.

2. On a rimmed baking sheet, put the tomatillos, whole serrano chile, and garlic, and grill on high for 5 minutes before blackening and softening begins. Then flip the tomatillos for about 5 minutes and roast the other hand (the tomatillos will change from green to olive green).

3. Allow it to cool, then move everything to a blender except for 1/2 of the chili pepper (including juices). Apply the cilantro and 1/4 cup of water and combine to the consistency desired. Taste, and, if desired, add extra chili pepper.

4. Dice the onion finely, then rinse under cold water as well as shake to eliminate excess humidity. Combine with the tomatillo mixture along with the salt in a serving bowl. If required, taste and add additional salt.

Easy Roasted Green Beans

Prep Time: 5 minutes

Cook Time: 15 minutes

Yield: 4

Ingredients

1 tablespoon olive oil

1-pound green beans

¼ teaspoon fresh ground black pepper

3/4 teaspoon kosher salt

1/2 lemon

1/4 teaspoon garlic powder

1/3 cup sliced or slivered almonds

Directions

1. Preheat the oven to 450 degrees Celsius.

2. Wash that green beans and cut the ends off.

3. Combine the beans with the kosher salt, olive oil, and fresh black ground pepper in a bowl. Line a parchment paper baking sheet, then place the beans mostly on the pan and roast for around 13 to 15 minutes, till just tender and lightly browned (before they get too dark brown).

4. Meanwhile, over medium heat, toast the almonds in the small dry frying pan, constantly stirring until toasted, around 5 minutes. Remove and chop from the heat.

5. Add squeezes of lemon juice and sprinkle with almonds when the beans are done roasting. Immediately serve.

Lemon Yogurt Sauce (+ Go Green Bowls)

Prep Time: 15 minutes

Cook Time: 20 minutes

Ingredients

2 cups dry quinoa

For the quinoa

1 teaspoon kosher salt

2 tablespoons olive oil

3 green onions

2 to 3 tablespoons fresh herbs (we used basil and chives)

Fresh ground pepper

Juice of 1 large lemon (use one of the lemons from the sauce)

For the lemon yogurt sauce

1 medium garlic clove

Peel of 1 1/ 2 lemons

3 tablespoons olive oil

1 cup Stonyfield Organic Whole Milk Yogurt

2 tablespoons capers

2 tablespoons tahini

1/2 teaspoon kosher salt

For the bowl

1 head broccolini (optional)

2 heads broccoli

1 tablespoon olive oil

1 bunch Tuscan kale

Fresh ground pepper

1/2 teaspoon kosher salt

Pepitas (optional)

8 cups fresh salad greens

Directions

1. Cook the quinoa (or use our quinoa system for the Instant Pot): Rinse the quinoa under cold water using a strainer, then fully drain it. Place the quinoa and three cups of water in a saucepan. Bring it to a boil, then bring the heat to a low level. Stir once, then boil where the water is only bubbling, changing the heat for around 17 to 20 minutes if necessary, until the water is fully absorbed (check by pulling back the quinoa with a fork to see if water remains).

2. Remove from the oven, cover the pot and allow 5 minutes for the quinoa to steam. Then, with a fork, fluff the quinoa and stir in the olive oil and kosher salt.

3. Meanwhile, cut the herbs, slice the green onion thinly, and add the lemon juice.

4. Stir in the basil, green onion, lemon juice, and pepper when the quinoa is done. Taste, and if necessary, add additional salt.

5. For the lemon yogurt sauce: Cut the peel of 1 1/2 lemons in very large pieces with a vegetable peeler (dig into the lemon with the peeler so that it comes off in large strips). Break it in half with the garlic. On a baking sheet, put the lemon zest and garlic and broil for about 5 minutes till the edges of the lemon peel begin to brown. Remove from the oven and slice roughly. Then mix the minced lemon peel and garlic with both the yogurt, olive oil, capers, and kosher salt in the bowl of an immersion blender (or handheld blender or food processor) and blend until creamy. Refrigerate before it's used (can store refrigerated for a few days).

6. For broccoli and kale: If used, chop the broccoli and broccolini. Chop and scrap the kale. Heat the olive oil in one big skillet over medium heat. Stir in the vegetables, salt, and pepper and saute for 1 minute. Add 1/4 of a cup of water and cook until the water evaporates and the broccoli is bright green and soft around 3-5 minutes. If required, taste and add additional salt. Place that fresh salad greens in the bowls and cover them with quinoa for serving. Then apply the mixture of broccoli and kale and drizzle with the lemon yogurt sauce. Sprinkle, if using, with pepitas.

Green Pea Soup with Chive Flowers

Prep Time: 20 minutes

Cook Time: 15 minutes

Yield: 4

Ingredients

2 thick slices whole-grain rye bread, cut into small cubes

1 tablespoon extra-virgin olive oil

Fresh chives with blossoms for garnish

Sea salt and freshly ground pepper

10 ounces fresh or frozen peas

2 3/4 cups vegetable stock

3/4 cup full-fat plain yogurt

1/4 teaspoon wasabi powder or paste (optional)

Finishing oil for drizzling (we used olive oil)

Directions

1. Over medium heat, heat the olive oil in a small skillet. In the oil, toss the bread cubes, turn with a tong or a heat-resistant spatula to toast on all sides for about 4 minutes. With salt and pepper, season. To cool, move to a plate. (You can do these up to one day in advance; just be sure to cool and store them in an airtight container completely.)

2. From the chives, pull the chive blossoms and chop the green shoots.

3. Heat the stock until simmering over high heat in a large soup pot. Add the peas and cook for 8 to 10 minutes, until bright green and just cooked. Remove from the heat and use an immersion blender or pass the soup to the blender in batches for approximately 3 minutes to process until smooth. Add (if used) the wasabi and season with salt and pepper. Add the yogurt and process it for 2 to 3 minutes until smooth and slightly creamy. Return to a pot and keep warm until you are ready to eat over a low flame.

4. In cups, ladle the broth, cover with croutons, and drizzle with olive oil. Season with pepper and generously scatter the chopped chives and their blooms over the end. Serve it sweet.

Spinach Meatballs with Feta

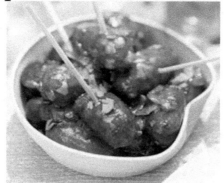

Prep Time: 15 minutes

Cook Time: 25 minutes

Yield: 2 to 4

Ingredients

2/3 cup crumbled feta cheese

14 ounces baby spinach or 9 ounces frozen, cooked spinach, thawed

1 egg

1 tablespoon mixed dried herbs

1/4 cup olive oil (for cooking, optional)

1/2 cup oat flour (process 1/2 cup rolled oats in a food processor or blender) or bread crumbs

2 tablespoons unsalted butter or extra virgin olive oil

10 ounces dry spaghetti (gluten-free, if necessary)

1 medium zucchini, shredded

2 tablespoons soy sauce or tamari

Freshly ground pepper

5 ounces cherry tomatoes, halved

Directions

1. When using fresh baby spinach, add a tiny splash of water to a big saucepan. Place and cover with a lid over the medium-low sun. Cook for 3 to 5 minutes, until wilted, then rinse under cold running water. To extract as much liquid as possible, squeeze the spinach over the drain, then chop coarsely and set aside. (Tip: it helps to minimize prep time by using frozen spinach; next time, we'll try that.)

2. Mix the feta, dried herbs, a generous amount of black pepper, the egg, and crumbles of oat flour or bread together in a medium cup. Stir in the chopped spinach, then scoop the mixture into heaping tablespoons and roll them into balls. Approximately 20 balls you can receive. You can either put them on a baking sheet lined with nonstick parchment paper and bake for 20 to 25 minutes in an oven preheated to 3500F or fry them in 2 batches over medium heat, in 2 tablespoons of oil per batch, turning 3 to 5 minutes on each side until golden. (Tip: We tried both ways, and it was easiest to find the baked version!)

3. Let the pasta boil, then drain.

4. Return the pasta from the heat to the tub, then whisk in the butter, tamari, or soy sauce, and the shredded zucchini. Toss and serve with halved cherry tomatoes.

Perfect Avocado Smoothie

Prep Time: 5 minutes

Cook Time: 0 minutes

Ingredients

1 large green apple

1/2 ripe avocado

1 cup baby spinach or kale, loosely packed (or other chopped greens)

1 banana

1 cup frozen pineapple chunks

1/2 cup water

1 tablespoon lemon juice

10 ice cubes

Directions

1. Pit the avocado into the blender and scoop one-half of the flesh out. Chop the fruit, and leave the skin on it. Break the banana into bits, then put both of them in the mixer. Add water and the leaves of the baby kale. Blend until perfectly smooth.

2. Add the ice, lemon juice, and frozen pineapple or mango. Blend until smooth again. Eat immediately, or store in a sealed jar for 1 to 2 days; shake to re-integrate if it separates.

Easy Vegan Tacos

Prep Time: 10 minutes

Cook Time: 20 minutes

Ingredients

2 tablespoons olive oil

1 1/2 cups green lentils

1 teaspoon garlic powder

1 teaspoon cumin

Fresh ground pepper

3/4 teaspoon kosher salt

For the tacos

2 green onions

8 One Degree sprouted organic corn tortillas

Salsa verde (purchased or homemade)

1/2 small green cabbage

Avocado or pickled jalapenos, optional

Creamy Cilantro Sauce, to serve

Directions

1. Soak the cashews for at least 30 minutes for the Creamy Cilantro Sauce while making the rest of the recipe (for a high-speed blender), or if you think of it, soak them overnight or in the morning. The better, the longer! (The sauce could also be made ahead of time, see instructions in the recipe for cilantro sauce!).

2. Put the lentils with 6 cups of warm water in a pot. Bring to a low boil, then boil until only al dente for around 15 to 20 minutes (taste often to assess doneness). Drain, and apply the olive oil, cumin, garlic powder, and kosher salt to the mixture.

3. Slice the green onions thinly. Slice the cabbage thinly. Chop the avocado if desired.

4. Make the Smooth Cilantro Sauce, in the meantime.

5. In compliance with the package instructions, warm the tortillas. (We usually char our own on an open flame, but with the One Degree tortillas, that's not the preferred method.) Cover the tortillas

with lentils, green onions, green cabbage, broken cilantro leaves, salsa verde, and cilantro drizzle to eat.

Chicken Fajita Lettuce Wraps

PREP TIME - 15 mins
COOK TIME - 30 mins
TOTAL TIME - 45 mins

Ingredients

2.0 bell peppers (thinly sliced into strips)

lb chicken breast (thinly sliced into strips)

tsp fajita seasoning

tsp olive oil

6.0 leaves romaine heart

tbsp fresh lime juice

1/4 cup non-fat Greek yogurt (optional)

Directions

• Wraps of Chicken Fajita Lettuce

1. To preheat. Preheat the 400 °F ovens to

2. Merge. Combine all the ingredients in one large plastic bag and seal (excluding Romaine). Mix well to cover uniformly.

3. PREP. Empty the contents of the bag on a baking sheet lined with foil and bake for 25-30 minutes until the chicken is thoroughly cooked.

4. You serve. Serve on Greek yogurt-topped Romaine leaves (if desired).

Nutrition

Protein: 40.0 g

Calories: 180.0 kcal

Cholesterol: 80.0 mg

Carbohydrates: 2.0 g

Fiber: 2.0 g

Fat: 5.0 g

Sugar: 5.0 g

Sodium: 300.0 mg

Low-Carb Baked Ricotta Cheesecake

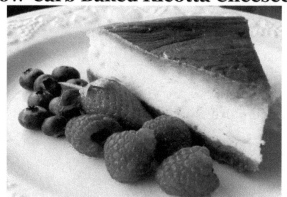

PREP TIME 10 mins

COOK TIME 25 mins

TOTAL TIME 35 mins

Ingredients

2 eggs

1 tsp vanilla extract

2 cups ricotta cheese (low-fat)

Directions

• Low Carb Baked Cheesecake Ricotta

1. To preheat. Preheat the oven to approximately 355°F/180°C

2. Mix the ricotta cheese and the vanilla extract together. If needed, add a sweetener.

Uh, 3. Beat. Mix the eggs gradually, and continue to beat together until the texture is smooth.

Oh, 4. Spoon. Spoon four ramekin dishes with the batter, then bake in a preheated oven (around 20-25 minutes).

5. You serve. Serve it with warmth!

Nutrition

Protein: 16.9 g

Calories: 206.0 kcal

Fat: 12.0 g

Carbohydrates: 6.7 g

Sugar: 0.7 g

Sodium: 186.0 mg

Blue Ribbon Blueberry Muffins

PREP TIME 15 mins

COOK TIME 30 mins

TOTAL TIME 45 mins

Ingredients

2 cups all-purpose flour

2 tsp baking powder

3/4 tsp salt

1 tbsp cinnamon

1/2 cup butter one stick. Make sure it's softened.

2 large eggs

1 1/2 tsp vanilla extract

1/2 tsp almond extract

1/2 cup milk

Directions

1. PREP. Preheat the oven to 375°C. Spray with non-stick spray on your muffin tin and line it with liners.

2. Merge. In a mixing bowl, whisk in the flour, baking powder, cinnamon, and salt.

3. For around 2 minutes, beat the sugar and butter together. Add the eggs one at a time until mixed, making sure to beat well after each one. The vanilla and almond extracts are then added.

4. Combine the dry mixture progressively into the wet one, making sure to mix well after each cup or so. Add in the blueberries to the batter and use your spatula to gently fold them in.

5. Bake until golden for approximately thirty minutes.

6. You serve. With a little bit of butter, enjoy soft or make-ahead and freeze up to 3 months. Enjoy!

Creamy Decadent Cashew Milk

PREP TIME 6 hrs
COOK TIME a few seconds
TOTAL TIME 6 hrs

Ingredients

1 cup raw cashews

4 cups water

2 tsp vanilla

1/2 tsp salt

2 dates

2 tsp vanilla

Directions

Creamy Decadent Milk Cashew

1.Enable your cashews and dates to soak up overnight for about 6 hours. You can skip this step if you are really in a hurry and have a powerful blender.

2. When the water is clear, drain your cashews and dates.

3. In your blender, combine all the ingredients, plus 4 cups of water, and mix.

4. To make thicker milk, add less water or more cashews to the mixture. Discard the cashew pulp or set aside for another recipe.

Nutrition

Fat: 9.0 g

Calories: 144.0 kcal

Protein: 12.0 g

Fiber: 4.0 g

Serving Unit: cup

Serving Amount: 1

Blueberry Buttermilk Pancakes

PREP TIME 10 mins

COOK TIME 20 mins

TOTAL TIME 30 mins

Ingredients

1 1/2 cup whole milk

4 tbsp white vinegar

2 cups all-purpose flour

4 tbsp sugar

2 tsp baking powder

1 tsp baking soda

1 tsp salt

2 eggs

4 tbsp melted butter + 1/2 tbsp unmelted

2 cups blueberries

1/2 tbsp butter, for the pan

Directions

Pancakes with Blueberry Buttermilk

Combine the vinegar and milk and let it sit for 1-2 minutes (this is the "buttermilk").

Whisk the flour, sugar, baking powder, baking soda, and salt together. Whisk the dry ingredients with the egg, milk, and butter until mixed.

Add 1/2 tbsp of butter to a non-stick pan over medium heat.

In the hot skillet, pour about 1/3 of a cup of batter and spread it (this will be thick). Arrange the pancake with the blueberries on top. Cook until little bubbles are seen on top, and the edges start to become solid. Flip and cook until the pancakes have risen, are fluffy, and cooked through for another 1-2 minutes.

Nutrition

Protein: 12.0 g

Carbohydrates: 75.0 g

Calories: 505.0 kcal

Fiber: 4.0 g

Fat: 16.0 g

Sugar: 24.0 g

Sodium: 635.0 mg

The Best-Ever Steak Marinade

PREP TIME 5 mins

COOK TIME a few seconds

TOTAL TIME 2 hrs

Ingredients

1/3 cup soy sauce

1/2 cup extra virgin olive oil

1/2 cup red wine vinegar

1/2 cup Worcestershire sauce

3 tbsp minced garlic

3 tbsp fresh chopped basil

1-1/2 tbsp dried parsley flakes

1 tsp fresh ground pepper

Instructions

The Best-Ever Steak Marinade

Combine all ingredients in a bowl. You can also blend them in a blender if desired.

Cook Put desired meat into a 13x9 inch pan and pour the marinade over the meat. Cover, and refrigerate for up to 8 hours. Cook meat as desired.

Nutrition

Carbohydrates: 6.0 g

Calories: 150.0 kcal

Protein: 2.0 g

Fat: 14.0 g

Sugar: 2.0 g

Sodium: 679.0 mg

Peanut Butter Protein Power Balls

PREP TIME 5 mins

COOK TIME a few seconds

TOTAL TIME an hr

Ingredients

1 cup coconut flour

1 cup peanut butter (can substitute with any nut butter or allergy-friendly alternative.)

1/4 cup chocolate chips

1/2 cup honey (or maple syrup)

1/4 cup flax seeds (can sub with hemp seeds.)

1/4 cup chia seeds (can sub with hemp seeds.)

Instructions

Peanut Butter Protein Power Balls

Mix. Combine wet and dry ingredients in a bowl

Spoon. Use a spoon and form into 24 balls (about 1 tablespoon size)

Freeze. Freeze 1 hour.

Serve. Enjoy!

Nutrition

Carbohydrates: 10.7 g

Calories: 121.0 kcal

Protein: 4.0 g

Fat: 7.5 g

Sugar: 4.8 g

Lean and Green Salad Recipes

Steamed Beans Tuna Salad Recipe

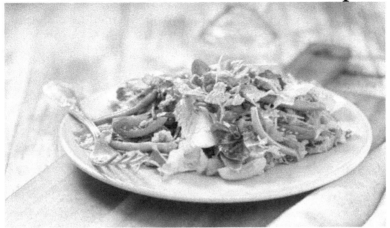

Ready in: 15 mins

Yield: 4 Servings

1 Lean, 3 Greens, 1 Fat, 3 Condiments

Ingredients

2 cups green beans, steamed

3 tablespoons balsamic vinegar

5 eggs, cooked/boiled

2 teaspoons of garlic powder

1 cup plum tomatoes, quartered

6 cups mixed greens

4 teaspoons canola oil

2 cans tuna in water, drained (about 7 ounces each)

1/4 teaspoon ground black pepper

Lemon wedges, optional

Instructions

Slice your boiled eggs and set them aside.

Add the vinegar, oil, and garlic in a small bowl. Mix until well combined.

Arrange your choice of mixed greens in a bowl. Layer the steamed beans, tomatoes, egg slices, and tuna.

Drizzle with oil mixture.

Serve with a sprinkle of black pepper and lemon wedges if desired.

Enjoy!

Nutritional Facts per Serving

351 calories; 12g carbs; 36g protein; 15.9g fat.

Shrimp Romaine Salad

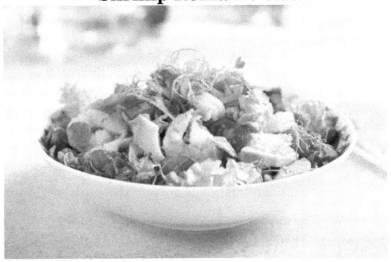

Ready in: 30 mins

Yield: 4 Servings

1 Leaner, 2 Fats, 3 Green, 3 Condiments

Ingredients

2 pounds shrimp, peeled and deveined

1 garlic clove

1 cups plum tomatoes, whole

2 scallions, white part only

1/2 tablespoons canola oil

1 teaspoons dried oregano

6 green olives, pitted and halved

2 lemons, juiced

1 avocado, pitted and diced

1/2 cup chopped cilantro

2 cups romaine lettuce, wash, torn, and chopped

Sea salt and ground black pepper to taste

Instructions

Preheat your oven to broil.

Bring a medium pot of water to a boil.

Add the shrimp to the boiling water and cook for 3 minutes until pink.

Remove shrimp from the heat, drain, and set aside to cool.

Combine the tomatoes, garlic, scallions, and oil in a sheet pan, stir and then broil in the oven for 7 minutes or the outside skin is charred.

Remove pan and allow to cool completely.

Once cooled, remove the core from the tomatoes, skin from the garlic, and root from the scallions. Place in a blender and blend briefly.

Transfer the blended mixture to a bowl. Add in the pitted olive, diced avocado, lemon juice, chopped cilantro, and shrimp, season with salt and pepper to taste, and then mix until combined.

Pour over romaine lettuce.

Enjoy!

Nutritional Facts per Serving

348 calories; 13g carbs; 49.4g protein; 12g fat.

Caesar Salad with Lemon Mayo Dressing

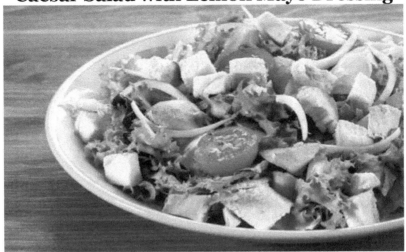

Ready in: 45 mins

Yield: 4 Servings

1 Lean, 3 Condiments, 3 Green, 1 Fat

Ingredients

For the Lemon Mayo Dressing

1 1/2 teaspoons lemon juice

1 tablespoon light mayonnaise

1/2 teaspoon Dijon mustard

1 teaspoon garlic powder

1/4 teaspoon each of salt and pepper

1 tablespoon shredded cheddar cheese

1 tablespoon canola oil

For the Salad

4 ounces zucchini, chopped

2 ounces chopped eggplant

6 cherry tomatoes, halved

1/4 cup shredded Parmesan cheese

1 pound grilled chicken breast, sliced or shredded

1 tablespoon fresh chopped cilantro

5 cups lettuce

Instructions

Preheat the oven to 400 F.

Roast the eggplant and zucchini on a greased baking sheet over medium heat until tender.

Combine all the dressing ingredients in a mixing bowl.

In another large bowl, combine the zucchini, cilantro, eggplant, tomatoes, lettuce, and parmesan.

Serve drizzled with dressing and grilled chicken.

Enjoy!

Nutritional Facts per Serving

379 calories; 58g protein; 13g fat; 8g carbs.

Easy Mashed Avocado Ranch Salad

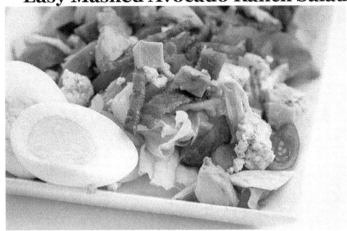

Ready in: 20 mins

Yield: 2 Servings

1 Leaner, 3 Green, 2 Condiments

Ingredients

1/2 avocado, cubed, divided

4 cups spring mix

1/2 pound cooked turkey bacon, sliced

1 cup cherry tomatoes, quartered

½ red onion, thinly sliced

2 hard-boiled eggs, sliced

1/4 cup low-fat, plain Greek yogurt

1 teaspoon dry ranch mix

1 teaspoon crushed pepper flakes

Instructions

Divide the spring mix among your serving bowls.

Add the bacon, sliced eggs, onions, a part of the cubed avocado, and tomatoes to each bowl.

Add the remaining part of the avocado to a blender and blend until smooth. Add in the yogurt, ranch mix, and a little water in the blender. Blend again until incorporated.

Top each salad bowl with the avocado mixture and a sprinkle of crushed pepper flakes.

Enjoy!

Nutritional Facts per Serving

280 calories; 32g protein; 16g fat; 28g carbs.

Avocado Shrimp Salad

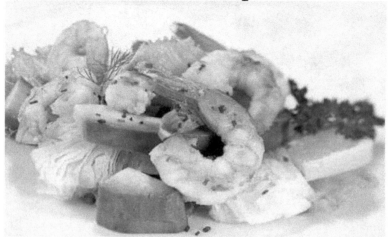

Ready in: 20 mins

Yield: 2 Servings

1 Lean, 2 Green, 2 Healthy Fats

Ingredients

1 large avocado, diced

14 oz cooked shrimp, peeled and deveined

1/3 cup green onion

1/4 cup jalapeno, de-seeded, diced

2 tablespoons lime juice

1/2 red bell pepper, sliced

1 teaspoon canola oil

1 tablespoon chopped parsley

A pinch of seas salt

1/8 teaspoon ground black pepper

Instructions

Add the onion, lime juice, oil, salt, and pepper to a re-sealable bag. Shake to combine and allow them to marinate for about 7 minutes.

Meanwhile, combine the shrimp, tomato, bell pepper, and avocado in a bowl and toss. Add the onion mixture to the bowl and stir again.

Add in the parsley and toss to combine.

Taste and add more salt and or pepper as needed.

Serve.

Enjoy!

Nutritional Facts per Serving

400 calories; 44g protein; 20g fat; 18g carbs.

Dill and Tomato Salmon Salad

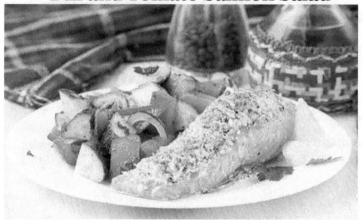

Ready in: 30 mins

Yield: 4 Servings

Ingredients

1 Lean, 3 Green, 3 Condiments

2 cups sliced cucumber

1 cup cherry tomatoes, halved

1/4 teaspoon salt

1/4 teaspoon black pepper

1/2 cup fresh dill, chopped

1/4 teaspoon smoked paprika

1/4 cup vinegar

1 1/2 pounds salmon

Instructions

Preheat your oven to 350 F.

Combine the sliced cucumber, tomatoes, vinegar, dill, salt, and pepper in a bowl.

Season the salmon on both sides with paprika and a little salt and place on a foil-lined baking sheet.

Roast until internal temperature reaches 145 F.

Serve salmon with salad.

Have fun!

Nutritional Facts per Serving

358 calories; 6g carbs; 36g protein; 21g fat.

Salmon with Garlic Lemon Asparagus

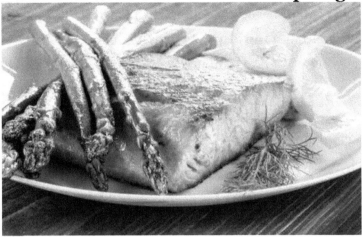

Ready in: 25 mins

Yield: 4 Servings

1 Lean, 3 Green, 3 Condiments

Ingredients

1 1/2 pounds salmon

1/4 teaspoon salt

1/4 teaspoon pepper

1/4 teaspoon ground coriander

1/4 teaspoon dried thyme

1/4 teaspoon parsley

1/2 teaspoon garlic powder

1 1/2 pounds asparagus, tough ends trimmed

1/4 cup grated Parmesan cheese

Lemon slices

Cooking spray

Instructions

Preheat oven to 400 F.

Combine the herbs and salt and pepper in a small bowl. Rub the mixture on both sides of the salmon.

Lightly spray the top of the salmon with cooking spray.

Place salmon in the center of a foil-lined, lightly greased baking sheet. Top with lemon slices.

Combine the Parmesan and garlic powder in another bowl. Arrange the asparagus around the salmon.

Lightly spray with cooking oil and sprinkle with Parmesan mixture.

Bake for about 18 minutes or until cooked through.

Enjoy!

Nutritional Facts per Serving

323 calories; 40.7g protein; 14g fat; 8g carbs.

Main Dish and snack Recipes

Instant Pot Pulled Pork

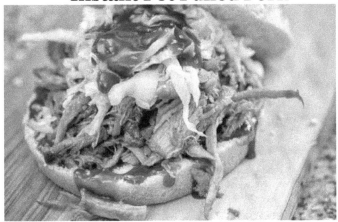

Ready in: 1 hr 20 mins

Yield: 4 Servings

1 Lean, 3 Green, 3 Condiments

Ingredients

2 pounds pork tenderloin, cut into two

1 (12-oz) can diet root beer

3 cups green cabbage, shredded

1/2 cup plain reduced-fat Greek yogurt

1 tablespoon apple cider vinegar

1 tablespoon lemon juice

1/2 teaspoon salt

3/4 teaspoon Dijon

3/4 cup sugar-free BBQ sauce

Ingredients

Spray the instant pot with cooking spray.

Set pot to Saute mode and cook pork for about 6 minutes or until browned, flipping halfway through.

Add in the root beer, secure the lid, and close the pressure valve. Set to 60 minutes at High Pressure.

Release pressure naturally before opening.

While the pork is cooking, combine the remaining ingredients in a bowl, mix well.

Discard liquid from the instant pot, transfer the cooked pork to a cutting board or bowl, and shred pork with two forks.

Transfer shredded pork pieces into a bowl, add in the BBQ sauce, and mix to combine.

Serve.

Nutritional Facts per Serving

405 calories; 12g fat; 47g protein; 17g carbs

Lime-Marinated Broccoli Pork Chops

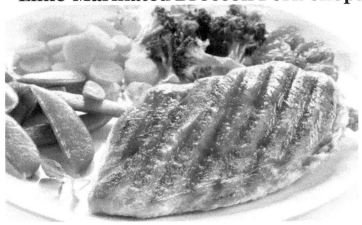

Ready in: 45 mins

Yield: 2 Servings

1 Lean, 3 Green, 3 Condiments

Ingredients

2 tablespoons lime/lemon juice

1 teaspoon extra virgin olive oil

2 cloves garlic, minced

1/4 teaspoon cinnamon

1/4 teaspoon coriander

1/4 teaspoon paprika

1 packet sugar substitute, optional

Salt and pepper to taste

1 pound raw, boneless pork loin chops

1 bunch broccoli, chopped

½ cup steamed green beans, optional

1/4 cup Parmesan cheese, shredded, optional

Instructions

Combine the first eight ingredients in a resealable bag. Add in the pork chops and shake vigorously to combine.

Set aside to marinate for at least 30 minutes.

Meanwhile, heat your grill to medium-high.

In a medium pot, heat water until boiling. Add chopped broccoli and allow to steam until tender-crisp.

Drain, cover, and set aside to keep warm.

Remove pork from the marinade, discard marinade, and grill pork for about 6 minutes per side or until internal temp reads 155 F.

Divide broccoli and pork chops between two serving plates. Top each plate with shredded Parmesan cheese and serve with steamed green beans if desired.

Enjoy!

Nutritional Facts per Serving

320 calories; 51g protein; 30g fat; 8g carbs.

Cauliflower Pork Medallion

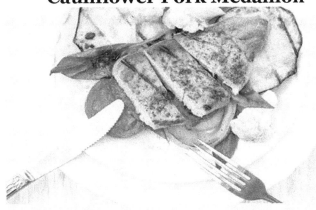

Ready in: 50 mins

Yield: 4 Servings

1 Lean, 3 Green, 3 Condiments

Ingredients

1/4 cup grape tomatoes, cut into halves vertically

1 tablespoon fresh thyme leaves

1 tablespoon fresh basil, chopped

1 teaspoon olive oil

2 teaspoons garlic powder

1/4 teaspoon sea salt

1/4 teaspoon ground black pepper

1 head cauliflower

1 1/2 pounds pork tenderloin, cut into 1/2-inch thick medallions

2 tablespoons poultry seasoning

¼ cup fresh chopped parsley

Instructions

Preheat your oven to 425 F.

Combine the tomato halves, oil, thyme, basil, garlic, and a pinch each of salt and pepper. Mix well.

Place the tomato halves cut-side up on a parchment-lined baking sheet and roast in the oven for 40 minutes.

Meanwhile, cut the cauliflower lengthwise through the core into 1/2-inch slices. Place the slices on a separate baking sheet with parchment paper, season with a pinch of salt and pepper, and spray with cooking spray.

Roast the cauliflower steaks for 30 minutes.

Preheat your grill. Rub pork with poultry seasoning and grill for 4 minutes, flipping halfway through until internal temperature reads 145 F.

To serve, place pork medallions on your serving platter, top with cauliflower steaks and roasted tomatoes. Garnish with a sprinkle of chopped parsley if using.

Have fun!

Nutritional Facts per Serving

302 calories; 10g carbs; 43g protein; 10g fat.

Kale, Tomato, and Goat Cheese Muffins

PREP TIME 10 mins

COOK TIME 20 mins

TOTAL TIME a few seconds

Ingredients

1 cup liquid egg whites

9 large eggs

2 oz goat cheese crumbled

3/4 cup plain, low-fat Greek yogurt

10 oz kale

1/2 tsp salt

cooking spray

2 cups cherry tomatoes

Directions

Muffins for Kale, Tomato, and Goat Cheese

1. The preheating. Preheat the furnace to 375 °F

2. Whisk. In a big bowl, whisk together the eggs, egg whites, Greek yogurt, goat cheese, and salt.

3. Stir. Stir in the cherry tomatoes and the kale.

4. Prep and replenish. Lightly grease two muffin tins and evenly separate the batter between the 24 wells.

5. Bake. Bake, 20-25 minutes or until it comes out clean with an inserted toothpick.

Nutrition

Protein: 29.0 g

Carbohydrates: 11.0 g

Calories: 290.0 kcal

Fiber: 3.0 g

Fat: 15.0 g

Sodium: 320.0 mg

Avocado Toast with Egg

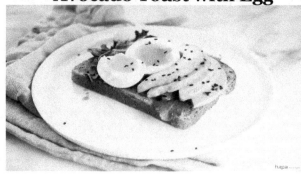

PREP TIME 15 mins

COOK TIME a few seconds

TOTAL TIME 15 mins

Ingredients

4 eggs

4 bread slices

Everything-But-The-Bagel Trader Joes Seasoning to taste

2 avocados

salt and pepper to taste

Directions

Avocado Egg Toast

1. Toast the four slices of bread as you mash the avocados together (as if you are making guacamole).

2. While toasting, mash the avocados together (as if you're making guacamole).

3. For avocados, add salt, pepper, and lemon juice (optional).

4. On the stove, fry eggs.

5. Spread the avocado mix on the toast and top it with the eggs. Enjoy, enjoy!

Nutrition

Carbohydrates: 13.5 g

Calories: 292.0 kcal

Protein: 8.1 g

Fat: 24.3 g

Sodium: 129.0 mg

Stuffed Zucchini

PREP TIME 15 mins

COOK TIME 1hr

TOTAL TIME 1hr

Ingredients

1 lb. pork or chicken sausage

3 zucchinis

1 clove minced garlic

1 cup dry breadcrumbs or cracker crumbs

3/4 cup grated parmesan cheese

1 32 oz jar tomato sauce (feel free to add extra spices to your taste)

shredded mozzarella cheese

1/2 cup

Directions

Stuffed Zucchini

1. Preheat to Preheat the oven to 350 degrees Fahrenheit

2. Trim the zucchini stems and vertically slice them. Scoop the seeds out and place them in a bowl.

3. Mix the sausage, garlic, breadcrumbs, and parmesan cheese with the seeds.

4. Cover the squash with the mixture of sausage and put in a baking pan of 9x13 inches.

5. To pour and cover, pour over the top of the zucchini spaghetti sauce and cover the plate with aluminum foil.

6. Bake, bake for about 45 minutes until the sausage is browned and cooked all the way through. Remove the foil and add the mozzarella cheese to the top.

7. Return, return to the oven and cook for about 15 more minutes until the cheese is melted.

Nutrition

Protein: 47.0 g

Carbohydrates: 46.0 g

Calories: 750.0 kcal

Fat: 34.0 g

Cholesterol: 80.0 mg

Sodium: 1170.0 mg

THM Cheeseburger Pie

PREP TIME 10 mins

COOK TIME an hr

TOTAL TIME an hr

Ingredients

1 tbsp onion powder

2 1/2 lb lean ground beef

3 cups cheddar cheese (grated)

1 1/2 tsp salt

1/2 cup mayonnaise

2 whole eggs

salt and pepper (to taste)

1/2 cup heavy cream

pickles

onions

tomato

jalapeno peppers

mustard

ketchup

Directions

THM Cheeseburger Pie

1. Cook the ground meat in a skillet over medium heat until brown. Drain the grease.

2. Add salt and onion powder.

3. Add the meat mixture in a casserole dish (or pie dish) and stir in half of the cheese.

4. Place a layer of any optional ingredients over the combination of meat and cheese (or skip for a more basic pie).

5. Whip the eggs, mayo, heavy cream, salt, and black pepper in another medium bowl.

6. Pour the mix over the ingredients, and finish with the remainder of the cheese.

7. Bake for 35 minutes at 350 degrees F.

Nutrition

Carbohydrates: 6.7 g

Calories: 544.0 kcal

Protein: 55.6 g

Fat: 31.8 g

Sugar: 2.4 g

Sodium: 821.0 mg

Grilled Shrimp Fajitas

PREP TIME 20 mins

COOK TIME 8 mins

TOTAL TIME 28 mins

Ingredients

bell peppers (color variety) (sliced into strips)

2.0 lbs medium shrimp (fresh is best, but frozen, thawed, then cleaned shrimp also works)

tbsp olive oil

limes (sliced)

large red onion (sliced into strips)

1/4 cup lime juice (key limes or Mexican limes work best)

8.0 tortillas (preferably corn)

tbsp olive oil

1/4 cup orange juice

tbsp shrimp fajitas seasoning blend

cloves garlic (minced)

tsp oregano

tbsp chili powder

tsp paprika

2.0 tsp cumin

2.0 tsp black pepper

2.0 tsp kosher salt

1/2 tsp onion powder

tsp garlic powder

1/2 tsp chipotle powder

Directions

Mix together the marinade fixings and add the shrimp. Throw to cover, cover with cling wrap and refrigerate for 15 minutes.

Sauté. In an enormous sauté container over high warmth, broil the chime peppers and onions in the oil until marginally limp and singed. Put in a safe spot.

Cook Shrimp

Barbecue. Preheat flame broil to 300°F and clean barbecue. Splash barbecue with cooking shower and flame broil shrimp, 1 to 2 minutes for each side contingent upon size. Move to a bowl and keep warm covered with aluminum foil.

Burner. In a huge flame broiling skillet over medium-high warmth on the burner. Add shrimp and then cook for 1 to 2 minutes for every side contingent upon size. Move to a bowl and then keep warm covered with the aluminum foil.

Mix. Add shrimp back to that skillet with vegetables and throw to mix and warm through.

Serve. Serve flame-broiled shrimp and vegetables with warm tortillas. Top with pico de gallo and guacamole (discretionary) and cut limes.

Slow-Cooker Pork

PREP TIME 10 mins
COOK TIME 6 hrs
TOTAL TIME 6 hrs

Ingredients

1 cup chicken broth

1 3-4lb pork roast

1/4 cup soy sauce

1/4 cup balsamic vinegar

2 tsp minced garlic

2 tbsp honey

2 tsp cornstarch

Directions

Moderate Cooker Pork

Spot broil in the lethargic cooker.

Consolidate remaining fixings (with the exception of cornstarch) in a 2-cup estimating cup. Whisk together and pour over a meal.

Cook on low 10-12 hours for that self-destruct, madly delicate sort of meat. (Or then again on high 6-8 hours.)

Pork Roast Gravy

Scoop and strain. Before serving, scoop out around 1/4 cup of the juice in the simmering pot and strain into an estimating cup.

Whisk in 2 tsp cornstarch. Include sufficient juice to make 1 cup.

Microwave on high for like 30 seconds and whisk once more. Pour sauce over meat before serving.

Nutrition

Saturated Fat: 2.0 g

Carbohydrates: 7.0 g

Calories: 331.0 kcal

Protein: 51.0 g

Cholesterol: 142.0 mg

Sugar: 5.0 g

Sodium: 635.0 mg

Slow Cooker Hawaiian Chicken

PREP TIME 20 mins

COOK TIME a few seconds

TOTAL TIME 20 mins

Ingredients

1 yellow onion chopped

2 lbs boneless skinless chicken breasts or chicken thighs

2 tbsp soy sauce

3 cups fresh pineapple diced

2 tbsp dark brown sugar

1 tbsp honey

1 tsp grated ginger

2 tbsp rice vinegar

1/2 cup your favorite BBQ sauce

1 tbsp minced garlic

1 1/2 cup diced bell pepper (orange, red, yellow mix) orange, red, yellow mix

1 tbsp cornstarch

1 tbsp water

sesame seeds for garnish if desired

parsley for garnish if desired

3 cups cooked white rice

Directions

Moderate Cooker Hawaiian Chicken

Using a skillet, brown the chicken on both sides for 3-5 minutes over high heat at that point and then add them to the slow cooker.

Add the pineapple and onion to the slow cooker.

Mix the nectar, soy sauce, brown sugar, ground ginger and garlic, and BBQ sauce into the sluggish cooker.

Cook on low for five hours or on the high for 3 hours.

Add the cornstarch to the tablespoon of water, mix, and add to the sluggish cooker with the chime peppers and let it cook an extra 30 minutes while you cook the white rice to go with your supper.

Serve over white rice with the parsley and sesame seeds.

Nutrition

Carbohydrates: 48.0 g

Calories: 230.0 kcal

Protein: 38.0 g

Fat: 12.0 g

Sugar: 12.0 g

Brunswick Stew

PREP TIME a few seconds
COOK TIME 3 hrs
TOTAL TIME 3 hrs

Ingredients

1 onion (quartered)

1 whole chicken (cut up)

1 tsp salt

2 ribs celery (diced)

16.5 oz white shoepeg corn

1/4 tsp pepper

1 lb canned tomatoes

10 oz frozen small butterbeans

1/3 cup ketchup

2 small potatoes (cubed)

1 tsp Worcestershire sauce

2-3 tbsp brown sugar

1/4 tsp marjoram

1/2 tsp Tabasco

2-3 tbsp butter

Directions

Brunswick Stew

Spot. Spot chicken in Dutch broiler and add enough water to cover well.

Season. Add onion, celery, salt, and pepper.

Bubble. Bubble until chicken falls off bones without any problem.

Cool. Eliminate chicken to cool and add corn, butterbeans, tomatoes, potatoes, ketchup, and earthy colored sugar.

Cook 2 hours, or until delicate.

Get ready. Eliminate chicken from bones and add to vegetables alongside Worcestershire, Tabasco, marjoram, and margarine.

Nutrition

Protein: 6.0 g

Carbohydrates: 28.0 g

Calories: 170.0 kcal

Fiber: 4.0 g

Fat: 5.0 g

Serving Amount: 1

Serving Unit: cup

Tom's Ultimate Cuban Sandwich

PREP TIME 20 mins

COOK TIME 35 mins

TOTAL TIME an hr

Ingredients

1 tbsp olive oil cooking spray

1 pork loin the smaller the better

1 1 take-and-bake French Baguette or other crusty bread. *

1 tsp garlic puree or two fresh garlic cloves

1/3 cup spicy brown mustard

1/2 cup mayonnaise

1/2 pound thinly sliced deli ham I use Boar's Head Branded Deluxe ham

1/4 tsp ground cumin

6 sandwich-sliced refrigerated dill pickles I use only Claussen pickles

8 slices swiss cheese

Directions

Tom's Ultimate Cuban Sandwich

Preheat stove to 350 degrees.

Place the pork midsection fat side up in a simmering container fixed with material paper or aluminum foil material. If the foil is utilized, shower with olive oil cooking splash.

Coat the top with the olive oil and rub with garlic. Liberally salt and pepper the whole outside of the pork.

Broil Roast for roughly 25 minutes for each pound or until the interior temperature comes to at any rate 165 degrees. Be mindful as not to overcook the pork broil. A marginally pink tone within is alright as long as the temperature is right.

Remove the cooked pork from the broiler and cool for 20 minutes.

Reset the boiler temperature to 425 degrees F.

Cut the loaf into four equivalent segments and cut each segment longways to shape four sandwich rolls.

Mix In one bowl, mix the mayonnaise, mustard, and cumin. Spread uniformly on each of the eight sandwich surfaces.

Cut Slice the meal pork into slight cuts and spot liberally on the base side of every one of the sandwiches.

Spot Place 2 cuts of swiss cheddar on top of the pork midsection cuts on each sandwich.

Spot Place 1/4 of the ham on the sandwich top side and top the ham with 1-1/2 dill pickle cuts each.

Toast Place each of the eight half-sandwiches open-looked on a heating sheet and toast on the center rack of the stove at 450 degrees for 8 minutes, until the cheddar is pleasantly softened. **

Cool Remove from the stove and permit to cool for 5 minutes.

Spot Place the topsides (ham/pickle) on the base side (pork/cheddar).

Cut Slice each sandwich fifty-fifty on a point.

Serve your Cubano with sides of new guacamole, dark beans, or potentially pot-cooked potato chips.

NOTES

*I like the LaBrea pastry kitchen loaves accessible in most supermarkets or the French rolls at Aldi and Whole Foods. A crusty bread, Italian bread portion, or Cuban bread would likewise work! **If you're, to a greater extent, a panini individual, you can utilize a panini press to toast the sandwiches!

Nutrition

Saturated Fat: 14.0 g

Carbohydrates: 37.0 g

Calories: 620.0 kcal

Fat: 39.0 g

Cholesterol: 110.0 mg

Protein: 34.0 g

Fiber: 3.5 g

Serving Amount: 1

Serving Unit: sandwich

Sugar: 5.0 g

Sodium: 640.0 mg

Tangy Fried Chicken Sandwich

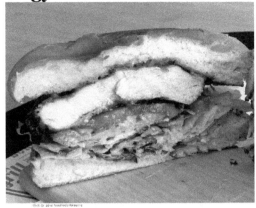

PREP TIME 15 mins

COOK TIME an hr

TOTAL TIME an hr

Ingredients

2 eggs

2 cups flour

1.5 tbsp pepper

2 tbsp hot sauce

2 tbsp Cajun seasoning

1 1/2 tbsp salt

vegetable or canola oil (Fill pot a third of the way up) for frying

ketchup to taste

2 tbsp honey

4 chicken breasts can use more if you have extra batter.

1 jar pickled jalapeños

1 package bacon about 8 pieces.

Directions

•Tangy Fried Chicken Sandwich

1.Pour. Fill a huge pot about 33% of the path up with any high-temperature oil you have close by. (Canola, vegetable, or nut). Try not to utilize olive oil since it has a lower smoke point and may make the chicken taste harsh.

2.Heat. When your oil is in the pot, set the burner to medium-high warmth until oil arrives at a temperature of 350 degrees Fahrenheit.

3.Prep. While your oil is warming up, get one plate for your chicken and two dishes. In the principal bowl, we will make our hitter.

•Fried Chicken Batter

1.Mix. Break three eggs into the bowl, trailed by some buttermilk (or if you don't have buttermilk, one cup of milk, and add a little lemon juice. One lemon wedge should do the trick.) Next, add some hot sauce to your decision.

•Fried Chicken Dredge

1.Mix.

In your subsequent bowl, pour two cups of flour, one teaspoon of heating pop, dark pepper, garlic powder, salt, and any Louisiana-style preparing you end up having close by.

•Frying the Chicken

1.Dredge. Next is the muddled part. Plunge your chicken into the dig first, at that point into the hitter, and afterward back into the dig. This will make a crispier outside. This will get everywhere on your hands, so be ready for that

2.Fry. Now, your oil ought to be up to temperature, and our chicken is prepared. Presently the entirety of that is left is fricasseeing. Put a few bits of chicken in the pot immediately for around 12 minutes, flipping once. While your chicken is broiling, set your broiler to 375 degrees.

3.Bake. After your chicken is finished broiling, it is essential to place the chicken in the broiler for around 8-10 minutes to ensure it is totally cooked through.

•Bacon

1.Sauté. While your chicken is in the broiler, take a skillet and begin cooking your bacon. A few bits of thick-cut bacon are suggested for each sandwich.

2.Rest. When your bacon is cooked, remove your chicken from the stove and let it sit for 2-3 minutes.

•Buns

1.Toast.

Our last advance is seemingly the most significant, consistently toast your buns. Toasted buns are vital for the sandwich' s unbending nature. Spill the bacon oil out of the skillet and several cuts of spread into the container on medium-low warmth. When the margarine is liquefied, lay your buns face down and stand by until they are brilliant earthy colored.

•Sauce

1.Mix. If you feel the buns are toasted as you would prefer, it's an ideal opportunity to build your sauce and prepare for a get-together of the sandwich. In a little bowl, pour three solid spurts of sriracha, nectar, mayonnaise, and ketchup. When the proportion of toppings is; however, you would prefer, it is time to amass our sandwich.

•The Ultimate Sandwich

1.Assemble. First, add your chicken bosom, trailed by bacon, jalapenos, pickles, singed onions (discretionary), lettuce, and your decision of cheddar. At long last, add a solid serving of sauce to the top bun and prepare to delve in!

Nutrition

Saturated Fat: 2.0 g

Carbohydrates: 44.0 g

Calories: 650.0 kcal

Protein: 30.0 g

Fat: 25.0 g

Sugar: 2.0 g

Avocado Cauliflower Rice

Prep Time 5 minutes

Cook Time 15 minutes

Total Time 20 minutes

Servings 6 cups

Ingredients

1 tablespoon cooking fat (avocado oil, coconut oil, ghee...)

6 cups cauliflower rice

3 cloves garlic, minced

1 cup diced yellow onion (120 grams)

1 jalapeño, diced

2 large avocados, diced (300 grams)

1/2 cup packed cilantro, roughly chopped

2 1/2 tablespoons lime juice

salt and pepper, to taste

Directions

1. Heat a huge sauté container over medium warmth. Add oil and let it get hot. When hot, add diced onions and sauté for 5 minutes until clear, mixing occasionally. Add garlic and cook for one more moment. Add the cauliflower rice and let cook for 6-7 minutes, mixing at times until relaxed.

2. While the rice cooks, make the avocado pound. Add avocados, diced jalapeno, lime squeeze, and salt and pepper to a huge bowl and squash with a fork until consolidated; however, a little surface remaining part.

3. Once cauliflower rice is cooked to your inclination, eliminate it from heat. Add avocado mixture to cauliflower rice and mix well to combine. Mix in cilantro. Top more cilantro and jalapeño if wanted. Appreciate!

Broccoli Cheddar Soup

Prep: 15 mins

Cook: 50 mins

Total: 1 hr 5 mins

Servings: 8

Ingredients

salt and ground black pepper to taste

½ onion, chopped

1 tablespoon butter

¼ cup flour

¼ cup melted butter

2 cups chicken stock

2 cups milk

1 cup matchstick-cut carrots

1 ½ cups coarsely chopped broccoli florets

2 ½ cups shredded sharp Cheddar cheese

1 stalk celery, thinly sliced

Directions

•Step 1

Soften one tablespoon margarine in a skillet over medium-high warmth. Saute onion in hot margarine until clear, around 5 minutes. Put in a safe spot.

•Step 2

Whisk 1/4 cup softened margarine and flour together in an enormous pot over medium-low warmth; cook until flour loses its granular surface, adding 1 to 2 tablespoons of milk if important to hold the flour back from consuming, 3 to 4 minutes.

•Step 3

Progressively empty milk into flour mixture while whisking continually. Mix chicken stock into milk mixture. Bring to a stew; cook until flour taste is gone, and the mixture is thickened around 20 minutes. Add broccoli, carrots, sautéed onion, and celery; stew until vegetables are delicate, around 20 minutes.

• Step 4

Mix cheddar into vegetable mixture until cheddar dissolves. Season with salt and pepper to taste.

Nutrition Facts

Per Serving:

Protein 14.3g; 304 calories; fat 23g; carbohydrates 10.7g; sodium 624mg; cholesterol 70.5mg.

Zucchini Hash Browns

Ingredients

salt, to taste

2 zucchinis

⅓ cup fresh chives (15 g)

½ cup parmesan cheese (55 g), grated

¼ teaspoon garlic powder

1 teaspoon dried oregano

1 egg

¼ teaspoon black pepper

Directions

1. Preheat broiler to 400°F/200°C.

2. Using a case grater, grind the zucchini on the coarse side.

3. Transfer the ground zucchini to an enormous bowl and sprinkle it with salt. Mix the zucchini and put it in a safe spot for 20 minutes while the salt draws dampness from the zucchini.

4. Transfer the zucchini to an enormous kitchen towel and strain the overabundance fluid into a bowl.

5. Place the zucchini back into the bowl and throw in the chives, parmesan, oregano, garlic powder, dark pepper, and egg, and mix until all around consolidated.

6. Portion the zucchini mixture into six even hash earthy colored patties on a material-lined heating sheet.

7. Bake for 35 minutes until browned.

8. Cool the hash browns for 10-15 minutes to set.

9. Serve with wanted plunging sauce.

10. Enjoy!

Chicken satay with peanut sauce

prep time: 2 HOURS 30 MINUTES

cook time: 20 MINUTES

total time: 2 HOURS 50 MINUTES

Ingredients

Kosher salt and freshly ground black pepper, to taste

2 tablespoons reduced sodium soy sauce

1/4 cup coconut milk

1 1/2 teaspoons turmeric

2 1/2 teaspoons yellow curry powder

1 tablespoon freshly grated ginger

3 cloves garlic, minced

1 tablespoon fish sauce

1 tablespoon brown sugar

1 tablespoon canola oil

2 pounds boneless, skinless chicken thighs, cut into 1-inch chunks

FOR THE PEANUT SAUCE

1 tablespoon reduced sodium soy sauce

3 tablespoons creamy peanut butter

2 teaspoons brown sugar

1 tablespoon freshly squeezed lime juice

1 teaspoon freshly grated ginger

2 teaspoons chili garlic sauce, or more, to taste

Directions

1. To make the nut sauce, whisk together peanut butter, soy sauce, lime juice, earthy colored sugar, bean stew, garlic sauce, and ginger in a little bowl. Speed in 2-3 tablespoons water until wanted consistency is reached; saved.

2. In a medium bowl, consolidate coconut milk, soy sauce, curry powder, turmeric, garlic, ginger, earthy colored sugar, and fish sauce.

3. In a gallon size Ziploc sack or huge bowl, consolidate chicken and coconut milk mixture; marinate for in any event 2 hours to expedite, turning the pack sporadically.

4. Drain the chicken from the marinade, disposing of the marinade.

5. Preheat flame broil to medium-high warmth. String chicken onto sticks. Brush with canola oil; season with the salt and pepper to taste.

6. Add sticks to flame broil, and cook, sometimes turning, until the chicken is totally cooked through, arriving at an interior temperature of 165 degrees F, around 12-15 minutes.

7. Serve quickly with nut sauce.

Parmesan Baked Zucchini

prep time: 10 MINUTES

cook time: 20 MINUTES

total time: 30 MINUTES

Ingredients

2 tablespoon chopped fresh parsley leaves

1/2 cup freshly grated Parmesan

4 zucchinis, quartered lengthwise

1/2 teaspoon dried oregano

1/2 teaspoon dried thyme

1/4 teaspoon garlic powder

1/2 teaspoon dried basil

2 tablespoons olive oil

Kosher salt and freshly ground black pepper, to taste

Directions

1. Preheat broiler to 350 degrees F. Coat a cooling rack with nonstick splash and spot on a heating sheet; put in a safe spot.

2. In a little bowl, consolidate parmesan, thyme, oregano, basil, garlic powder, salt, and pepper, to taste.

3. Place zucchini onto arranged preparing sheet. Shower with olive oil and sprinkle with Parmesan mixture. Spot into the broiler and prepare until delicate, around 15 minutes. At that point, cook for 2-3 minutes, or until fresh and brilliant earthy colored.

4. Serve quickly, decorated with parsley, if wanted.

Garlic Butter Sauteed Zucchini

PREP 5mins

COOK 5mins

TOTAL 10mins

Makes 4 servings

Ingredients

1 tablespoon butter

1 1/4 pounds chopped zucchini (2 medium)

Salt and fresh ground black pepper

1 tablespoon minced garlic (3 cloves)

Dash fresh lemon juice or red wine vinegar, optional

1/4 cup fresh grated parmesan or pecorino cheese, optional

1 scallion, thinly sliced

Directions

You can cut the zucchini any way you would like into, half-moons or chop it into bite size pieces.

Liquefy the margarine in a wide skillet over medium-high warmth. Add the zucchini and garlic and cook, blending every so often until the zucchini is seared in spots and delicate, 3 to 5 minutes.

Season with a touch of salt and dark pepper. Mix in the scallions and cheddar, if utilizing. Serve promptly with a spritz of lemon juice.

Teriyaki Halibut

Ingredients

Dash of salt and/or pepper (optional)

2-1/4 cups cabbage, chopped

7 oz raw halibut (should yield one 6-oz cooked serving)

2 tsp teriyaki sauce

1 cup (1 small) zucchini, chopped

1/2 tsp cayenne pepper (optional; for less "heat," use 1/2 tsp paprika instead, or eliminate)

1 tsp olive oil

Directions

Fish: Sprinkle halibut with cayenne pepper or paprika and treat with teriyaki sauce. Sear on tin foil 4" under preheated grill 7 minutes. Eliminate from stove and enclose by tin foil until prepared to serve (this will keep on cooking halibut). Vegetables: Chop up zucchini and cabbage. Sauté olive oil, zucchini, and cabbage in a skillet until somewhat earthy colored. Season with salt and pepper to taste if wanted. Spot on plate and serve halibut on top of vegetables.

Savory cilantro salmon

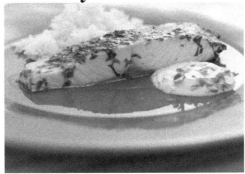

Total Prep: 1hr 25mins

SERVES: 2

Ingredients

1 tablespoon fresh lime juice

1 1/2 cups fresh cilantro leaves

1/2 teaspoon salt

1/2 teaspoon ground cumin

10 ounces salmon fillets

1 dash hot pepper sauce

1 medium red bell pepper, seeded and

1 medium yellow bell pepper, seeded and sliced

Directions

• To get ready marinade, in a food processor, join cilantro, juice, cumin, salt, hot sauce, and 1/4 cup water. Puree until smooth.

• Transfer marinade to gallon-size sealable plastic sack; add salmon. Seal pack, crushing out air, go to cover salmon. Refrigerate 60 minutes, turning pack sometimes.

• Preheat stove to 400. Shower 9-inch heating dish with a nonstick splash.

• Arrange pepper cuts in a single layer in arranged dish; prepare 20 min, turning peppers once.

•Drain salmon, dispose of the marinade. Spot salmon on top of pepper cuts, prepare, turning salmon once, 12-14 moment until fish chips effectively when tried with a fork.

• 6 Points per serving (1 salmon filet).

Crab and Asparagus Frittata

Prep: 20 mins

Cook: 10 mins to 12 mins

Servings: 6

Yield: 1 frittata

Ingredients

⅓ cup milk

8 eggs

1 tablespoon snipped fresh tarragon or basil

¼ cup grated Parmesan cheese

¼ teaspoon salt

½ teaspoon black pepper

¼ cup chopped onion

2 teaspoons olive oil

1 ½ cups bias-cut fresh asparagus (1-inch pieces) *

3 cloves garlic, minced

bottled hot sauce (optional)

6 ounces fresh or canned lump crab meat, drained, flaked, and cartilage removed

2 tablespoons water

2 tablespoons snipped fresh Italian parsley

⅓ cup bottled roasted red sweet peppers, drained and chopped

Directions

•Step 1

Preheat grill. In a bowl, whisk together the initial six fixings (through salt).

• Step 2

Warmth oil in an enormous broiler-proof skillet over medium warmth; add the onion and garlic. Cook 2 minutes. Add asparagus and the water. Cover and cook for 4 to 5 minutes or until asparagus is delicate. Channel and dispose of any fluid excess in the skillet.

• Step 3

Equitably sprinkle the crab and cooked peppers over asparagus. Pour egg mixture over the vegetables and crab in skillet. Cook over medium warmth. As mixture sets, run a spatula around edge of skillet, lifting egg mixture so uncooked bitstreams under. Keep cooking and lifting edges until the egg mixture is practically set (the surface will be wet).

• Step 4

Spot skillet under the grill 4 to 5 crawls from heat. Sear 1 to 2 minutes or until the top is simply set. (Or, on the other hand, preheat stove to 400°F; heat around 5 minutes or until the top is set.)

• Step 5

Cut into wedges. Sprinkle with parsley and present with hot sauce.

Grilled Chicken with Peanut Sauce

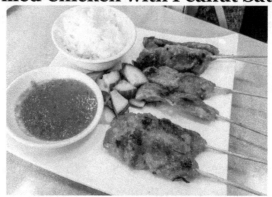

PREP TIME: 10 MINUTES

COOK TIME: 10 MINUTES

MARINADE TIME: 10 MINUTES

TOTAL TIME: 30 MINUTES S

SERVINGS: 4 PEOPLE

Ingredients

2 garlic cloves finely chopped or grated

4 boneless, skinless chicken breasts

3 Tablespoons olive oil

1 Tablespoon lime juice

Fresh cilantro chopped (for garnish)

Salt and pepper to taste

PEANUT SAUCE:

⅓ cup water

1/2 cup peanut butter

1/4 cup cilantro leaves

1 lime juiced

2 Tablespoons avocado or canola oil

2 garlic cloves

1 Tablespoon fish sauce

2 Tablespoons sriracha

2 teaspoons brown sugar

1 Tablespoon soy sauce

Directions

Warmth barbecue to medium.

Cut every chicken bosom fifty-fifty on a level plane into two equally thick parts.

Whisk together garlic, lime juice, and olive oil in an enormous bowl. Season to taste with salt and pepper. Add chicken and go pieces to altogether cover. Let marinate 10 minutes, and as long as 30 minutes, at room temperature.

In the meantime, make the nut sauce.

In a food processor or blender, join all fixings and interaction until smooth, adding more water if expected to thin.

Barbecue chicken until sautéed and cooked through, 2 to 3 minutes for every side.

Move chicken to a platter. Spoon nut sauce over the chicken and sprinkle with cilantro, if wanted. Offer excess nut sauce as an afterthought.

NOTES

DO AHEAD: Peanut sauce can be made three days ahead.

Main Dish Recipes

Cheeseburger Soup

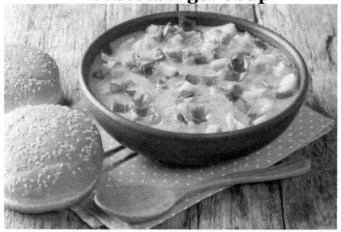

Ready in: 50 mins

Yield: 4 Servings

1 Lean, 3 Green, 1 Fat, 3 Condiments

Ingredients

3 cups of water

1 pound lean ground beach

1 cup celery, diced

1 teaspoon parsley

1/2 onion, chopped

2 cups peeled and diced potatoes, optional

1 teaspoon dried basil

1 (14.5-oz) can diced tomatoes

Salt and pepper to taste

1 1/2 teaspoons plain, low-fat Greek yogurt

1 bunch spinach, torn

1 cup low-fat goat cheese, grated

Instructions

Brown the beef in a large soup pot.

Add the chopped onion, parsley, basil, and celery and saute for a couple of minutes until tender.

Remove beef from the heat and then drain off any excess fat.

Add in the water, tomatoes, potatoes (if using), yogurt, salt, and pepper. Cover and simmer for 20 minutes on low until potatoes are fork-tender.

Add in the spinach and cook for 2 minutes until wilted.

Serve topped with cheese.

Have fun!

Recipe Note: Nutritional facts do not include potatoes.

Nutritional Facts per Serving

401g calories; 44.2g protein; 20.3g fat; 11g carbs.

Cajun Pork Chops and Spinach Salad

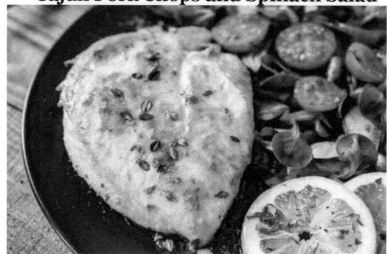

Ready in: 30 mins

Yield: 4 Servings

1 Lean, 3 Greens, 3 Condiments

Ingredients

8 cups baby spinach

28-ounce pork chops

1 tablespoon Cajun seasoning

1 cup fresh tomatoes, chopped

1 lemon, juiced

1/2 teaspoon each of salt and ground black pepper

Lemon wedges for garnish

<u>Instructions</u>

Season the pork chops with the Cajun seasoning, 1/8 teaspoon salt, and 1/8 teaspoon pepper.

Set aside to marinate for about 25 minutes. (The longer the better)

Cook the pork in a preheated oven at 450 F for 10 minutes.

Meanwhile, heat the water in a pot. Add in the spinach and cook until wilted.

Transfer the spinach to a bowl. Add in the tomatoes, lemon juice, the remaining salt, and pepper.

Serve pork chops with spinach salad and lemon wedge(s) by the side.

Enjoy!

Nutritional Facts per Serving

301 calories; 12.3g carbs; 28g protein; 16g fat.

Creole Shrimp Lettuce Wraps

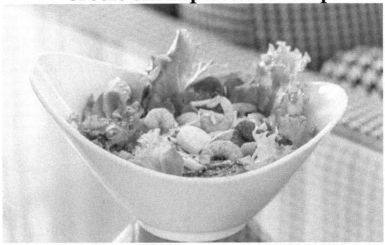

Ready in: 35 mins

Yield: 4 Servings

1 Leanest, 2 Fats, 3 Greens, 3 Condiments

Ingredients

12 romaine lettuce leaves

2 pounds raw shrimp, peeled and deveined

4 teaspoons avocado oil

1 tablespoons creole seasoning

1 avocado, cubed

1 cup plain, low-fat Greek yogurt

Juice of 1 lemon

1/4 teaspoon turmeric

A pinch of sea salt

1 1/2 cups diced tomatoes

1/2 onion, chopped

1 tablespoon chopped fresh cilantro leaves

1 jalapeno pepper, chopped and seeds removed

Instructions

Place the shrimp, turmeric, creole seasoning, and salt in a zip-lock bag.

Shake the bag vigorously. Heat the oil in a skillet. Add the shrimp to the hot oil in a single layer.

Cook for 2 minutes, flip over and cook another 2 minutes until the shrimp are cooked through and pinky. (You may need to work in batches). Set aside.

Next, Place the avocado, yogurt, and half of the lemon juice in a blender and blend until smooth. Set aside.

Combine the tomatoes, onion, cilantro, jalapeno, and the remaining lemon juice in a bowl. Mix well.

Divide the shrimp among the lettuce wraps.

Top each wrap with avocado mixture and tomato salsa.

Serve topped with more cilantro if desired.

Enjoy!

Nutritional Facts per Serving

351 calories; 39g protein; 15.1g fat; 16.9g carbs.

Pesto Zucchini Nutty Noodles

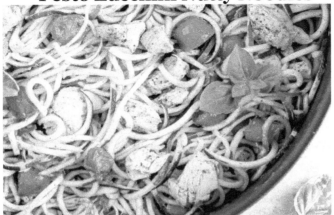

Ready in: 25 mins

Yield: 4 Servings

1 Leaner, 3 Greens, 1 Healthy Fat, 3 Condiments

Ingredients

1/3 cup low-fat ranch dressing

1/2 cup parmesan

1/4 cup chopped cashew nuts

2 teaspoons almonds

1/2 cup chopped fresh basil leaves

2 medium zucchinis, spiralized

1 1/2 pounds grilled skinless and boneless turkey breast, sliced

2 cups grape tomatoes, sliced into cubes

1/2 teaspoon crushed red pepper flakes

Instructions

Combine the ranch dressing, 1/4 cup parmesan, basil, cashew nuts, and almonds in a blender and process until smooth.

Lightly grease a skillet and cook the zucchini in the skillet over medium heat for 4 minutes or until just tender.

Stir in the blended mixture and the remaining parmesan, and then remove from the heat.

Add in the tomatoes and grilled turkey.

Serve garnished with a sprinkle of pepper flakes.

Enjoy!

Nutritional Facts per Serving

412 calories; 43.4g protein; 17.1g fat; 14g carbs.

Chipotle Chicken & Cauli Rice Bowl

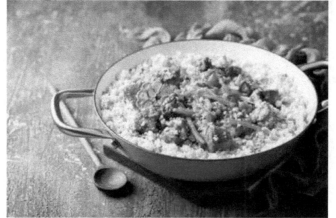

Ready in: 35 mins

Yield: 4 Servings

1 Leaner, 3 Greens, 1 Fat, 3 Condiments

Ingredients

1 canned chipotle pepper in adobo sauce

1 cup low-fat shredded Mozzarella

1 (14 oz) can fire-roasted diced tomatoes

3/4 teaspoon cumin

3/4 teaspoon dried oregano

4 cups riced cauliflower

1 1/2 pounds boneless chicken breasts

1/2 cup salsa

Sea salt to taste

Instructions

Add the diced tomatoes, salsa, chipotle, cumin, oregano, and salt to a food processor and process until smooth.

Place the chicken breasts in your instant pot and pour the blended mixture over the chicken.

Secure the lid and close the valve. Adjust the instant pot to cook at High Pressure for 20 minutes, and then naturally release the pressure.

Transfer the chicken to a bowl. Shred the chicken, return the shredded pieces to the pot and toss to combine with the sauce.

In the meantime, place the cauliflower rice in a microwave and microwave according to package directions.

When ready to serve, divide the cauliflower rice among your serving bowl. Top each bowl with chicken and mozzarella.

Enjoy!

Nutritional Facts per Serving

393 calories; 16g fat; 48g protein; 13g carbs.

Classic Stuffed Bell Peppers

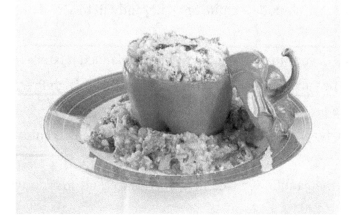

Ready in: 30 mins

Yield: 2 Servings

1 Lean, 3 Greens, 3 Condiments

Ingredients

4 large bell peppers (any color)

1 pound ground deli roast beef

2 tablespoons chopped onions

1 cup shredded low- fat mozzarella cheese

1/4 cup low-sodium chicken broth

2 garlic cloves, minced

1 cup sliced cremini mushrooms

3 tablespoons reduced-fat cream cheese

Instructions

Preheat oven to 400 F.

Cut a thin slice from the stem end of each bell pepper to remove the top of the pepper.

Remove the seeds and ribs, rinse the peppers, and set aside.

Saute the onion and garlic in broth in a large skillet over medium-high heat until the onions are translucent, 4-5 minutes.

Add the mushrooms, and continue to cook until tender.

Stir in the beef and heat through for about 4 minutes. Remove the skillet from the heat and mix in the cream cheese.

Line the inside of each pepper with 1/8 cup of mozzarella and an equal amount of beef mixture, and then top off with remaining cheese.

Bake for 18-20 minutes or until peppers are tender and the cheese is melted.

Serve with bean salad for a filling lunch.

Enjoy!

Nutritional Facts per Serving

292 calories; 32g protein; 14.7g fat; 6.8g carbs.

Lean and Green

Prep: 10 mins

Total: 10 mins

Servings: 1

Yield: 1 serving

Ingredients

1 banana

1 cup fresh spinach

4 hulled strawberries

½ green apple

⅓ cup whole milk

4 (1 inch) pieces frozen mango

1 teaspoon honey

1 scoop vanilla protein powder (Optional)

Directions

Step 1

Mix spinach, banana, apple, strawberries, mango, milk, protein powder, and nectar together in a blender until smooth.

Cook's Note:

Milk estimation can be adapted to favored thickness.

Nutrition Facts

456 calories; protein 43.3g; carbohydrates 66.9g; fat 4.9g; cholesterol 20.6mg; sodium 272.8mg.

Jalapeno Green Smoothie

Prep: 5 mins

Total: 5 mins

Servings: 2

Ingredients

2 cups baby spinach

2 bananas, broken into chunks

½ teaspoon chopped jalapeno pepper, or to taste

1 cup frozen mango chunks

1 cup water, or as desired

Directions

Step 1 Layer banana, spinach, mango, and jalapeno pepper in a blender; add water and mix until smooth, adding more water for a slenderer smoothie.

Nutrition Facts

Per Serving:

166 calories; protein 2.6g; carbohydrates 42.1g; fat 0.7g; sodium 30.1mg.

Green Monster Smoothie

Prep: 5 mins

Total: 5 mins

Servings: 1

Yield: 1 smoothie

Ingredients

½ cup fat-free plain yogurt

1 cup fat-free milk

1 tablespoon natural peanut butter

1 banana, frozen and chunked

1 cup ice cubes (Optional)

2 cups fresh spinach

Directions

Step 1 Mix milk, yogurt, banana, peanut butter, spinach, and ice solid shapes until smooth.

Nutrition Facts

382 calories; protein 23.6g; carbohydrates 55.7g; fat 9.4g; cholesterol 7.4mg; sodium 328mg.

Maple Lemon Tempeh Cubes

Cook Time: 30 mins

Total Time: 30 mins

Ingredients

2–3 teaspoons coconut oil

1 package tempeh (I use LightLife's Three Grain)

2 teaspoons maple syrup

3 Tablespoons lemon juice

2 teaspoons water

1–2 teaspoons low-sodium tamari or Bragg's Liquid Aminos (optional)

1/4 teaspoon powdered garlic

1/4 teaspoon dried basil

fresh ground black pepper, to taste

Directions

Warmth stove to 400°. Cleave your square of tempeh into scaled-down squares. Warmth coconut oil in a non-stick skillet on medium-high warmth. When dissolved and hot, add tempeh and cook for 2-4 minutes on one side or until the tempeh turns a brilliant earthy-colored tone on the base. Flip the bits of tempeh and cook for another 2-4 minutes.

While tempeh is cooking, mix together the lemon juice, maple syrup, tamari, water, basil, garlic, and dark pepper. Pour mixture over tempeh and mix around to cover the tempeh. Sauté for 2-3 minutes, at that point, flip the tempeh and sauté another 1-2 minutes. The tempeh ought to be overall quite earthy colored on the two sides.

The tempeh is prepared to serve in the wake of sautéing; however, if you need the pieces a touch crunchier, place on a heating sheet and heat for 15-20 minutes in the stove. Eliminate from the broiler, plate, and serve.

Easy Bok Choy Stir-Fry with Tofu

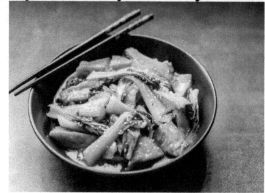

Prep Time: 15 minutes

Cook Time: 15 minutes

Total Time: 30 minutes

Ingredients

1 Tablespoon coconut oil

1 lb. of super-firm tofu (drained and pressed)

3 heads of baby bok choy, chopped into bite-size pieces

1 clove of garlic, minced

2 teaspoons maple syrup

5–6 Tablespoons low-sodium vegetable broth

1–2 teaspoons Sambal Oelek, or similar chili sauce

2 teaspoons Braggs liquid aminos or low-sodium tamari

½ – 1 teaspoon fresh ginger, grated

1 green onion/scallion, chopped

rice or quinoa, for serving

Directions

Wipe squeezed tofu off with paper towels, and cut into little reduced down pieces, about ½ inch thick. Warmth coconut oil on medium in a huge skillet. Add tofu and pan-fried food until delicately shaded. Around 5-6 minutes.

Add garlic and bok choy to the skillet. Sautéed food for around 1-2 minutes until the bok choy starts to shrink. The skillet will begin to dry out a piece; when this occurs, you'll need to add the vegetable stock just as all the leftover fixings (maple syrup, fluid amino, Sambal Oelek, scallion, and ginger). Keep pan-searing the mixture until all fixings are all around covered and the majority of the fluid vanishes, around 5-6 minutes.

Serve over quinoa or earthy-colored rice.

Healthy chicken pho with zucchini noodles

Prep Time: 10 minutes

Cook Time: 50 minutes

Total Time: 1 hour

Ingredients

10 cups of chicken stock

2 large chicken breasts, bone in

3-inch knob of ginger

1 large onion

4 whole cloves

2-star anise

1 tbsp coconut sugar

2 tbsp fish sauce

1/2 tsp black pepper

1 tsp sea salt

optional: 1/2 hot pepper, sliced

4 handfuls of bean sprouts

2 heads of bok choy

fresh basil

3 large zucchinis, spiralized on the smallest blade.

1 lime, cut into wedges

Directions

Preheat stove to 475 degrees F.

Strip onion and cleave down the middle.

Strip ginger and cut into three little lumps.

Spot on a preparing sheet and heat on the top rack for 25 minutes.

Flip onion and ginger part of the way through.

Include star anise and entire cloves in the most recent 5 minutes of heating to toast somewhat.

Spot stock in a huge pot and heat to the point of boiling.

When bubbling, include chicken bosoms and cook for 5 minutes.

Skim off the "filth" that buoys to the top and dispose of.

Eliminate chicken from the pot and put it aside to cool somewhat.

When the stove is done, slash up ginger and onions and add to stock.

Cleave chicken off the bone and add to stock.

I like to add the chicken bones once again into the stock to give it more profundity of flavor. However, this is discretionary.

Add toasted star anise and cloves, fish sauce, coconut sugar, salt, dark pepper, and hot pepper if utilizing to stock.

Bring stock a bubble and afterward lower warmth and let stew for 60 minutes.

Eliminate chicken bones if utilizing.

Add in bok choy and permit to wither.

Separation bean fledglings and zucchini noodles into four dishes and stop with soup.

Spot basil and lime wedge on top and serve.

If putting away for a few days, keep stock separate from bean fledglings and zucchini noodles, so they don't get soft.

Vegan Edamame Quinoa Collard Wraps

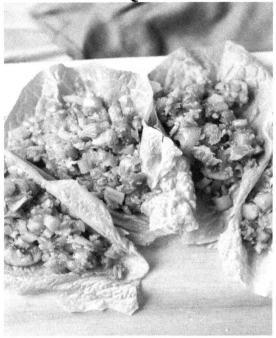

Prep Time: 15 mins

Cook Time: 0 mins

Total Time: 15 mins

Ingredients

For the wrap:

1/3 cup shelled defrosted edamame

1/4 cup grated carrot

2–3 large collard leaves

1/4 red bell pepper, chopped into thin strips

1/4 cup sliced cucumber

1/3 cup cooked quinoa

1/4 orange bell pepper, chopped into thin strips

For the dressing (you will have lots of leftovers):

1 cup cooked chickpeas

fresh ginger root, about 3 tbsp, peeled and chopped

4 tbsp rice vinegar

1 large clove of garlic

2 tbsp lime juice

2 tbsp low sodium tamari or coconut aminos

a few pinches of chili flakes

1/4 cup water

1 packet stevia (optional)

Directions

Set up the dressing first. In a food processor, join all fixings and puree until smooth. Fill a little bowl or holder and put it in a safe spot.

Lay the collard leaves on a level surface, covering each other to make a more grounded wrap.

Take 1 tbsp ginger dressing and mix it into the cooked quinoa.

Spoon the cooked quinoa onto the leaves, framing a straight level line on the end closest to you.

Follow with the edamame and all leftover veggie fillings.

Shower around 1 tbsp a greater amount of the ginger dressing up and over, at that point overlap the sides of the wrap internal towards one another. Crease the side of the wrap closest to you over the fillings; at that point, roll the whole wrap away from you to shut it down.

Jalapeño Chickpea Lentil Burgers with Sweet Mango Avocado Pico

PREP TIME15 MINUTES

COOK TIME10 MINUTES

TOTAL TIME25 MINUTES

Ingredients

1 - 15 oz can of chickpeas, rinsed and drained

1/2 cup dried red lentils, rinsed and drained

1 tsp chili powder

1 tsp ground cumin

1/2 cup packed cilantro

1 tsp sea salt, plus more to taste

1 jalapeno, de-seeded and finely chopped

2 garlic cloves, minced

1 red bell pepper, very finely diced

1/2 small red onion, minced

1/4 cup oat bran or oat flour, gluten-free if desired

1 large carrot, very finely chopped or shredded

Lettuce or Hamburger Buns, to place patty in

For pico:

1 ripe avocado, diced

1 large ripe mango, diced

1/2 cup chopped cilantro

1/2 small red onion, finely diced

sea salt, to taste

1/2 tsp fresh lime juice

Directions

To make mango avocado pico: Place all fixings in a bowl and mix to consolidate. Add salt to taste. A spot in cooler until prepared to serve.

Spot a medium pot over medium-high warmth, add lentils and 1/2 cups of water; heat water to the point of boiling, at that point cover, diminish warmth to low and stew lentils for around 10-15 minutes or until the fluid is consumed and lentils are extremely delicate and somewhat soft. Channel any abundance of water and put it in a safe spot.

Spot the chickpeas, cooked lentils, garlic, cilantro, ocean salt, cumin, and stew powder in a food processor and mix until the beans and lentils are smooth.

Move the mixture into a huge bowl. Mix in onion, jalapeno, red pepper, and carrot. Taste and change flavors as fundamental. Include oat grain a little at an at once into the mixture with your hands. You need to have the option to frame patties; however, you don't need an excess of oat wheat, or the burgers will self-destruct. So use however much you feel important. Since these burgers don't utilize an egg to tie them, you'll need to immovably shape the patties yet keep them pretty thick with the goal that they don't handily self-destruct. The gap into six equivalent parts and shape into thick patties with your hands.

Warmth skillet over medium-high warmth; include a 1/2 tablespoon of olive oil (at times, I showed the two sides of the burger with olive oil cooking splash as well). Spot a couple of burgers in an at once for a couple of moments on each side, or until brilliant earthy colored and fresh. Rehash with outstanding patties and keep on adding olive oil depending on the situation.

Spot patties in lettuce or in a bun and top with mango avocado pico.

Nutrition
Fat: 6.1g
Calories: 225kcal
Fiber: 12.7g
Carbohydrates: 34.9g
Protein: 9.6g
Sugar: 7.7g

Strawberry & Kale Slaw Chicken Salad with Poppyseed Dressing (GF)

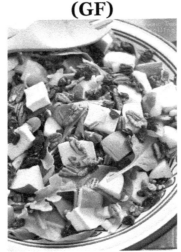

Prep time 20 mins

Total time 20 mins

Serves: 2

Ingredients

1 cup kale, chopped

1 cup strawberries, sliced

8 oz baked chicken breast, sliced (I just used salt and pepper to season)

¼ cup slivered almonds

For The Dressing:

2 teaspoons dijon mustard

1 tablespoon light mayonnaise

1 tablespoon apple cider vinegar

1 tablespoon olive oil

1 tablespoon agave nectar or raw honey

½ teaspoon lemon juice

¼ teaspoon garlic powder

¼ teaspoon onion powder

2 teaspoons poppyseeds

Directions

Whisk together dressing fixings until very much joined and set in the cooler to chill.

Heat chicken bosoms, cool, and cut.

Gap kale, slaw, and strawberries among two dishes.

Top with the cut chicken bosom (4oz each), and sprinkle with almonds.

Gap the dressing and shower over every serving of mixed greens.

Notes

*Costco conveys a Kale Slaw serving of mixed greens mix, which turns out impeccably for the base of this serving of mixed greens - you can likewise utilize the poppyseed dressing that comes in the plate of mixed greens mix if you lack as expected.

Nutritional Information

Serving size: ½ recipe Calories: 340 kcal

Shrimp, Broccoli, and Shitake Mushroom Stir Fry

Prep time 10 mins

Cook time 15 mins

Total time 25 mins

Serves: 4

Ingredients

Garlic cloves, minced – 2

Frozen shrimp – 1 lb.

Broccoli, chopped – 1 crown

Onion, chopped – 1

Corn starch – 1 tbs. + 2 tsp.

Shitake mushrooms, sliced – ¼ lb.

Rice vinegar – 1 tsp.

Soy sauce – 2 tbs.

Chicken stock – ½ cup

Brown sugar (or another sweetener) – ½ tbs.

Lemon juice – ½ tbs.

Grapeseed or canola oil – 2 tbs.

Shitake mushrooms, sliced – ¼ lb.

Broccoli, chopped – 1 crown

Lemon juice – ½ tbs.

Prep (can be done earlier in the day)

Onion, garlic, mushrooms, broccoli, – Chop as directed

Shrimp – Defrost shrimp. Rinse and dry with paper towels

Directions

Throw shrimp with one tbs. of corn starch and season with salt and pepper

Make the sauce by mixing soy sauce, vinegar, sugar, 2 tsp altogether. corn starch, and chicken stock

Warmth a wok over medium-high warmth. Add one tbs. Oil and afterward shrimp to warmed oil.

Saute shrimp until the outside is brilliant – it doesn't need to be cooked through as far as possible.

Return skillet to medium-high warmth and add remaining oil. Add garlic and afterward cleaved onions with a scramble of salt. Saute onions until mellowed, ~2 minutes

Add broccoli with a scramble of salt. Pan-fried food for 2 minutes and afterward adds cut shitake mushrooms, likewise with a scramble of salt.

Add shrimp back in not long after the shitakes. Push all fixings to the side of the skillet to frame a doughnut in the center. Give the sauce mixture a mix if corn starch has sunk to the base. Fill the focal point of the dish. Trust that mixture will obscure and bubble a great deal. At that point, throw to cover everything.

Cook until shrimp is done (you'll simply need to cut into a piece or take a chomp). Eliminate from warmth and add lemon juice. Season to taste with salt and pepper

Easy Honey Mustard Chicken Skillet

Prep Time10 minutes

Cook Time20 minutes

Total Time30 minutes

Ingredients

1 1/2 Tbsp Olive oil, divided

1/4 Cup Slivered almonds

1 Pound Grass-fed Chicken breast, cut into strips

1 Tbsp Fresh garlic, minced

2 Cups Asaparagus, chopped (about 1 large bunch)

4 Cup Zucchini, sliced (about 2 small)

For the sauce:

4 Tbsp Honey

1 Cup Reduced-sodium chicken broth

1 Tbsp Balsamic vinegar

1/4 Cup Dijon Mustard (make sure it's paleo friendly)

2 tsp Reduced-sodium soy sauce (gluten free if needed)

1 Tbsp Tapioca starch *

Sliced fresh basil, for garnish

Pinch of sea salt

Hot cooked rice or cauliflower rice, for serving

Directions

Warmth your stove to 400 degrees and line a little preparing sheet with material paper. Toast the almond in the broiler until they are light, brilliant earthy colored, for a couple of moments. Set aside.

Warmth 1 Tbsp of the olive oil in a huge skillet on medium/high warmth. Include the garlic and cook until brilliant earthy colored, pretty much one moment.

Turn the warmth down to medium and include the chicken bosom strips. Cook, blending now and then, until the pieces are not, at this point, pink inside. When cooked, move to a bowl and cover.

When the chicken has been eliminated, turn the warmth back up to medium-high, include the leftover oil, and let it heat. At that point, include the zucchini and asparagus. Cook, blending habitually until the veggies are daintily caramelized. Include the chicken pieces and cook for one moment or two.

In one medium bowl, whisk together all the sauce fixings, trying to truly disintegrate the custard. Add the sauce into the dish, mix, and heat to the point of boiling for one moment. Decrease the warmth to medium and stew until the sauce is overall quite thick, around 3-5 minutes.

Trimming with toasted almonds and basil and serve over quinoa or rice.

Nutrition

Carbohydrates: 28.1g, Calories: 335kcal, Fat: 5.5g, Protein: 31.2g, Polyunsaturated Fat: 0.5g, Saturated Fat: 0.7g, Sodium: 669mg, Monounsaturated Fat: 3.7g, Fiber: 4g, Potassium: 679mg, Vitamin A: 2400IU, Sugar: 21.6g, Calcium: 39mg, Vitamin C: 23.9mg, Iron: 1.4mg

Kale and broccoli salmon burgers

Prep Time: 45 mins

Cook Time: 10 mins

Total Time: 55 mins

Ingredients

1/2 cup almond meal (or old-fashioned oats or breadcrumbs)

1–15oz can wild salmon, drained + skin and bones removed

2 tbsp lemon juice

2 large eggs

1/2 tsp garlic powder

1/2 tsp salt

1/2 cup very finely chopped kale (stems removed)

Pepper, to taste

1/2 cup chopped onion

1/2 cup very finely chopped broccoli florets

1/2 cup finely chopped parsley (optional)

Directions

Spot depleted salmon in a huge bowl (I eliminate the skin and bones, yet that is discretionary).

Add eggs, almond dinner, lemon juice, salt, garlic powder, and pepper. Mix well to consolidate.

Include hacked veggies. Be certain they are cleaved into small pieces on the grounds that the burgers will self-destruct if there are huge lumps. Mix well (I utilized my hands).

Structure into five firmly stuffed patties. Spot on a plate fixed with foil or material paper and refrigerate for in any event thirty minutes.

When refrigerated, heat an enormous skillet splashed with oil over medium warmth. When hot, add burgers. Cook for 5-7 minutes for every side or until seared.

Crunchy Thai Kale Salad

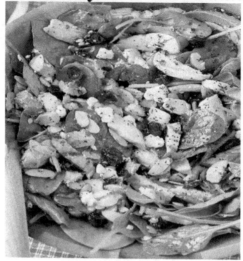

PREP TIME - 20 minutes

TOTAL TIME - 20 minutes

Ingredients

For the Salad:

1/2 cup thinly sliced carrots

4-5 cups packed curly or lacinato kale

1/4 cup cubed firm tofu (organic, non-GMO if possible)

3 small radishes* (thinly sliced)

1/2 Tbsp agave or maple syrup (or honey if not vegan)

1/2 Tbsp sesame oil

1 tsp lime juice

1 Tbsp sesame seeds (you'll have leftover)

3-4 Tbsp peanut sauce (for topping)

For the Peanut Sauce:

1 Tbsp soy sauce (tamari if gluten-free)

1/4 cup salted natural peanut butter (creamy or crunchy)

1/2 medium lime, juiced (1/2 lime yields ~1 1/2 Tbsp)

2-3 Tbsp brown sugar (or sub agave, maple syrup or honey if not vegan)

Hot water

1/2 tsp chili garlic sauce

Sriracha (optional // for a little heat)

Directions

Channel tofu by enveloping a towel and squeezing delicately. Let rest for 5 minutes. At that point, open up, shape, and throw in sesame seeds. If you don't care for crude tofu, look at this "Make Tofu Taste Good" formula! Simply overlook the sesame seeds, so they don't consume in the broiler.

Plan nut sauce by whisking all fixings together aside from the water. At that point, include 1 Tbsp heated water a little at an at once. Taste and change flavors on a case-by-case basis.

Add kale to an enormous mixing bowl and sprinkle with lime juice, toasted sesame oil, and agave. Back rub with hands for one moment to fuse fixings and relax the leaves.

So, Add kale to the serving plate or bowl and top with cut radishes, carrot, and sesame-tofu. Shower with nut sauce and serve right away. Extras store well, even softly dressed. Will keep refrigerated for up a few days, however best when new.

Notes

*You can sub 1/4 cup cut red onion instead of 3 little radishes.

*Nutrition data is a harsh gauge for one plate of mixed greens and does exclude the entirety of the dressing – only 3-4 Tbsp.

Nutrition (1 of 1 servings)

Calories: 528: Carbohydrates: 59g, Protein: 22g, Fat: 26g, Saturated Fat: 3g, Trans Fat: 0g, Cholesterol: 0mg, Sodium: 1100mg, Fiber: 9g, Sugar: 26g

Tempeh & green vegetables with tangy peanut sauce

Ingredients

Veggies:

½ cup frozen spinach

3oz tempeh, cubed

½ cup broccoli

½ cup green bell pepper, chopped

¼ cup un-shelled edamame

¼ cup chopped yellow onion

½ clove garlic, minced

¼ cup low-sodium vegetable broth

Sauce:

1 Tbsp low-sodium soy sauce

1 Tbsp unsalted peanut butter

¼ tsp garlic powder

1 Tbsp apple cider vinegar

Directions

Empty vegetable stock into a dish over low warmth. Join tempeh, spinach, chime pepper, broccoli, onion, edamame, and garlic in the container and cook until vegetables are delicate, and the vegetable stock has been absorbed. In a different bowl while vegetables and tempeh are cooking, whisk together all sauce fixings; if wanted, add a touch of water for a slenderer consistency. Put sauce in a safe spot. When vegetables have completed the process of cooking, add the nut sauce and coat uniformly.

Spaghetti squash primavera

Prep Time 10 minutes

Cook Time 20 minutes

Total Time 30 minutes

Ingredients

2 tablespoons extra-virgin olive oil

1 Spaghetti Squash

1 onion, minced

2 garlic cloves, minced

1 cup grape tomatoes, quartered

1/3 cup sun-dried tomatoes, soaked in warm water for a few minutes, drained and then roughly chopped

1 head broccoli, sliced into bite-sized florets

4 asparagus, sliced thinly

1/2 teaspoon red pepper flakes, more to taste

1/4 teaspoon ground garlic powder

Fine sea salt, more to taste

Freshly ground pepper, more to tase

1 lb. organic boneless chicken breast, cooked as desired*

2 handfuls fresh organic spinach

Optional: 2 tablespoons parmesan cheese

10 shrimp, cooked**

Directions

1. Preheat stove to 375 °F.

2. Roast spaghetti squash.

3. Heat oil in a huge pot over medium-high warmth. Add garlic and onion and sauté for 3-5 minutes or until the onion begins to turn clear.

4. Add in sun-dried tomatoes, grape tomatoes, asparagus, broccoli, and flavors. Sauté for 3-5 minutes, or until broccoli and asparagus start to mellow.

5. Add in spaghetti squash and cook for 1-2 minutes.

6. Toss in spinach and cook just until the spinach starts to wither.

7. Place in wanted serving bowls and top with new parmesan, chicken, and shrimp. Serve warm.

Nutrition

Calories: 391; Sugar: 3.6g; Sodium: 320mg; Fat: 16.7mg; Carbohydrates: 9g; Fiber: 2g; Protein: 48g; Cholesterol: 217mg

Miso Vegetables & Tofu

Prep time: 10 minutes

Cook time: 20 minutes

Serves 4 - 6, plus leftover dressing.

Ingredients

1/4 cup sake

6 oz awase miso (or blend or equal parts white & red miso)

3 tablespoons sifted natural cane sugar

1/2 cup mirin

4 cups / 12 oz / 340 g bite-sized veggies (see headnotes)

red pepper flakes or shichimi tōgarashi, a big pinch or two

12 ounces / 340 g baked or grilled (or lightly pan-fried) firm tofu, cut into bite-sized pieces

Directions

Start the dressing first. Join miso, purpose, mirin, and sugar in a little pot. Heat just to the point of boiling, dial down the warmth, and stew tenderly for around 20 minutes or until it thickens a piece. In the end, mix in the red pepper drops, adding to taste. Eliminate from warmth and permit to cool.

Meanwhile, heat a pot of water to the point of boiling. Salt the water and whiten the vegetables momentarily, sufficiently long to bring some relief, close to a moment. I realized the broccoli might require 20-30 seconds longer to cook than the slight asparagus, so I added it to the pot first. Utilize your best judgment dependent on whatever vegetables you are utilizing. Channel and quickly run under virus water to stop the cooking. Channel well, you need to attempt to get however much water off the vegetables as could reasonably be expected.

In a huge serving bowl, delicately throw the vegetables until completely covered with 1/3 cup/80 ml of the miso dressing. Add the tofu and throw once more. Taste and add really dressing if you like; simply remember, this specific dressing is very solid and rich. Serve family-style or exclusively finished off with a smidgen more shichimi tōgarashi or a sprinkling of red pepper pieces.

Broccoli + Spiced Lentil Power Plate!

Savory Miso Broccoli

1 small bunch of broccoli (about 2-3 cups of chopped florets) – organic

1/2 tsp extra virgin olive oil

1 tsp tamari

1 1/2 Tbsp white miso paste

2-3 Tbsp nutritional yeast

1/4 cup water

pepper   to   taste

Toasty Spiced Lentils

1 can of cooked lentils, organic – drained and rinsed well

1/2 tsp extra virgin olive oil

2 small lemons, juiced

spices: any will work! I simply used some fine black pepper!

1/4 cup white onion, diced

2 Tbsp fresh flat leaf parsley, finely chopped

Tahini Sauce

1 tbsp lemon juice

1-2 tsp grade B maple syrup

1 Tbsp tahini

Other:

1 handful mixed greens

2-3 fresh orange slices

1/2 avocado, sliced

Directions

1. Open lentils and channel fluid from a can. Wash lentils in virus water well overall. Put in a safe spot.

2. Wash and slash your broccoli. Cleave onion and parsley and juice lemons.

3. Whisk together your miso base for the broccoli. Add the miso, water, and tamari to a cup and mix until diminished.

4. Warmth a huge skillet over high warmth. Add 1/2 tsp of olive oil. Add the broccoli and throw broccoli in an oil apiece. Add the miso-water mixture up and over the broccoli and cover with a skillet top. Permit the broccoli to steam and cook for around 1-2 minutes over high warmth. When the broccoli is just about delicate enough to serve, include the nourishing yeast. This will cover the broccoli and add a decent additional layer of appetizing flavor. Add a discretionary sprinkle of vinegar or lemon juice if the broccoli looks altogether too dry. You could likewise include another sprinkle of water if required and permit that to steam the broccoli further. Cook until all the broth has been absorbed and a pleasant covering coats your broccoli. Move hot broccoli to a serving plate.

5. No compelling reason to wash the skillet. Add a 1/2 tsp of olive oil and your lentils, flavors, and onion. Utilizing a spatula, scratch the sides of the skillet, so any extra "sauce" from the broccoli blends with the lentils. Include a sprinkle of lemon juice to help deglaze the container. Toast lentils for around 1-3 minutes over high warmth. Similarly, as the lentils appear to be done, include parsley and lemon juice. Serve lentils when they are toasted and practically become "fleecy" as the external skins toast up and within turns out to be delicate from the warmth.

6. Add your small bunch of greens to the plate, close to the broccoli. At that point, add the lentils up and over. Add the avocado and citrus and a couple of portions of newly slashed parsley too. Ultimately, whisk together your tahini sauce/shower and pour it up and over your plate as wanted.

Thai chicken zucchini noodles

PREP TIME 15 minutes

COOK TIME 8 minutes

TOTAL TIME 23 minutes

Ingredients

salt & pepper

1 chicken breast

1 large zucchini, peeled/spiralized (I used a julienne peeler)

1 tablespoon coconut oil

2 tablespoons cashews, chopped

1/4 cup cilantro, chopped

1 tablespoon peanut butter

1 carrot, chopped

1/2 tablespoon honey

1/2 lime, juiced

1/2 tablespoon fish sauce

2 tablespoons coconut cream from a can

1 clove garlic, minced

1 teaspoon ginger, minced

1/2 tablespoon jalapeno, minced

Directions

1. Heat a skillet over medium-high warmth and liquefy coconut oil.

2. Season chicken bosom with salt and pepper, and once hot, add to skillet.

3. Cook for around 3-4 minutes for each side until cooked through.

4. Remove from skillet and shred, put in a safe spot.

5. In a little bowl consolidate, peanut butter, lime juice, nectar, coconut cream, fish sauce, ginger, garlic, and jalapeno. Whisk together and then put in a safe spot.

6. Combine destroyed chicken in an enormous bowl with stripped/spiralized zucchini, cilantro, cashews, and carrots.

7. Pour the sauce in the bowl and throw to consolidate.

Healthy Green Bean Casserole

Prep Time: 20 minutes

Cook Time: 58 minutes

Total Time: 1 hour 18 minutes

Ingredients

Crispy Baked Onions

1/4 cup oat flour

2 medium onions, thinly sliced

1 teaspoon sea salt

2 tablespoons panko breadcrumbs (gluten-free, if needed)

Nonstick cooking spray

Green Beans and Sauce

1 cup unsweetened almond milk

½ cup cashews (soaked)

2 Tablespoons vegan butter

24 oz fresh green beans, rinsed, trimmed and halved

1 teaspoon sea salt

12 ounces baby bella mushrooms, trimmed and cut into 1/2-inch pieces

3 cloves garlic, minced

1 teaspoon ground pepper

2 Tablespoons oat flour

1/4 teaspoon ground nutmeg

1 teaspoon low-sodium tamari (or soy sauce)

1 cup vegetable broth

Directions

1. Add 1/2 cup cashews to a bowl with water for dousing. Let douse for in any event 30 minutes.

2. Preheat the broiler to 475°F.

3. Combine the onions, flour, panko, and salt in an enormous mixing bowl and throw to join. Coat a sheet container with a non-stick cooking splash and equally spread the onions on the dish. Spot the

skillet on the center rack of the broiler and prepare until brilliant earthy colored, roughly 25 minutes, throwing like clockwork. When done, eliminate from the broiler and put aside until prepared to utilize. Decrease broiler temperature to 375°F.

4. While the onions are cooking, set up your green bean mixture.

5. Bring some huge pot of water to a bubble. Add the beans and whiten for 5 minutes. Channel in a colander and promptly dive the beans into a huge bowl of ice water to stop the cooking. Channel and put aside in an enormous bowl.

6. Drain cashews and add to a blender with almond milk. Mix until smooth and velvety and put in a safe spot.

7. Melt the margarine in a huge skillet over medium-high warmth. Add the mushrooms, salt, and pepper and cook, infrequently blending for 4 to 5 minutes. Add the garlic and nutmeg and keep on cooking for another 1 to 2 minutes. Sprinkle the flour over the mixture and mix to join. Cook for one moment. Add the stock and tamari, stew for one moment. Decline the warmth to medium-low and add the cashew cream. Cook until the mixture thickens, blending incidentally, roughly 6 to 8 minutes.

8. Remove from the warmth and empty sauce into a huge bowl with the green beans and ½ cup of the fresh heated onions. Spot green bean mixture into an 8×8 heating dish and top with the leftover firm prepared onions. Spot into the broiler and prepare until bubbly and warm all through, roughly 15-20 minutes. Eliminate and serve right away

Dessert

Vanilla Chocolate Cheesecake

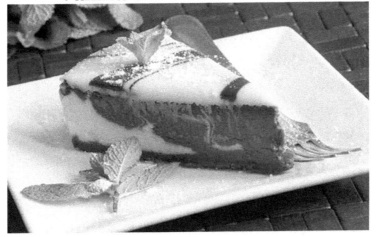

Ready in: 1 hr 10 mins

Yield: 1 Serving

1 Fueling, 1 Fat, 1/2 Lean, 3 Condiments

Ingredients

4 tablespoons cold water

2 sachets Optavia Essential Double Chocolate Brownie

1/2 tablespoon unsalted butter, melted

1 cups reduced-fat plain Greek yogurt

3 tablespoons light cream cheese

1 egg

2 teaspoons stevia

1/2 teaspoon pumpkin pie spice

1 teaspoon pure vanilla extract

1/8 teaspoon salt

1/2 teaspoon ground cinnamon

Instructions

Preheat your oven to 350 F.

Add the chocolate brownie, butter, and water to a bowl and mix well to combine.

Divide the mixture among two lightly greased mini springform pans. Press mixture into the bottom of the pans to form thin crusts and then bake for 15 minutes.

While baking, add the remaining ingredients to a medium bowl and mix until well incorporated, and then divide among the two pans.

Reduce oven temperature to 300 F and continue to bake for another 35 minutes or until the edges of the cheesecake turn golden brown and a toothpick inserted into the center comes out clean.

Remove from the oven and let cool for a couple of minutes before removing and slicing.

Enjoy!

Nutritional Facts per Serving

316 calories; 25g fat; 21g protein; 16g carbs.

Peanut Butter Cookies

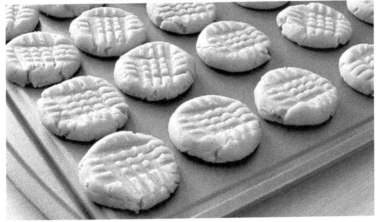

Ready in: 50 mins

Yield: 3 Servings (10-12 cookies)

1 Fueling, 1/2 Healthy Fat, 1/2 Condiment

Ingredients

4 sachets Optavia Peanut Butter Shake

1/4 teaspoon baking powder

1 egg

1/4 cup vanilla almond milk

1 tablespoon unsalted butter, melted

1/4 teaspoon pure vanilla extract

A pinch of sea salt

1 teaspoon ground cinnamon

Instructions

Preheat your oven to 350 F.

Combine the Peanut Butter and baking powder in a small bowl.

Add in the milk, egg, butter, and vanilla and stir to combine.

Place parchment on a cookie sheet and spray with cooking spray.

Divide dough evenly into 12 cookies.

Place cookie apart on a baking sheet.

Lightly grease a fork and use the back of the fork to flatten the cookies.

Sprinkle the top of each cookie with salt and cinnamon and then bake in the preheated oven for at least 10 minutes until set.

Serve and enjoy!

Nutritional Facts per Serving

98 calories; 4g protein; 6g fat; 4g carbs.

Almond Brownie Pie

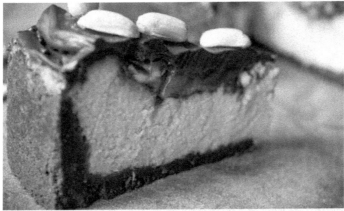

Ready in: 30 mins

Yield: 2 Servings

1 Fueling, 1 condiment, 1/2 Healthy Fat, 1 Optional Snack

Ingredients

2 sachets Optavia Decadent Double Chocolate Brownie

1/4 cup peanut butter powder

3 tablespoons liquid egg substitute

1/3 teaspoon baking powder

1/2 cup + 2 tablespoons unsweetened almond milk

1 teaspoon canola oil

Instructions

Preheat the oven to 350 F.

Combine the Chocolate brownie, egg substitute, 4 tablespoons milk, baking powder, and canola oil in a bowl and mix until it forms a batter.

Lightly grease a four-cup muffin tin and divide the batter among the four cups of the muffin tin, place in the oven and bake for about 20 minutes.

While the batter is baking, mix the peanut butter and the remaining milk in a small bowl.

Remove brownie pies from the oven and allow them to cool. Then slice each horizontally. Top one half of the pie with the peanut butter mixture and cover with the other half. Repeat for the remaining brownie pies.

Nutritional Facts per Serving

165 calories; 6g protein; 10g carbs; 9.4g fat

Cinnamon Cheese Sticks

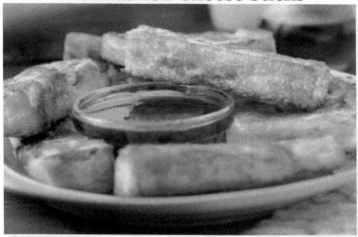

Ready in: 25 mins

Yield: 2 Servings

1 Fueling, 3 Condiments

Ingredients

2 sachets Optavia Essential Cinnamon Crunchy Cereal

6 tablespoons liquid egg substitute

2 tablespoons reduced-fat cream cheese

1/4 teaspoon ground cinnamon

Instructions

Place the Cinnamon Crunchy in a blender and blend until it forms bread-like consistency. Transfer mixture to a mixing bowl.

Add in the cream and egg substitute and mix to form a dough, and then form 6-8 sticks from the dough. Sprinkle with ground cinnamon.

Heat a lightly greased skillet over medium heat, and cook the sticks until and lightly browned.

Enjoy!

Nutritional Facts per Serving: 89 calories; 4.2g fat; 5.6g protein; 1.4g carbs.

CONCLUSION

It is clear to all that the longer you live a healthy lifestyle, the more chances you have to live a healthy and productive life! So, what does a healthy lifestyle mean?

The most important factor is that you need to eat a healthy, low fat diet. Because your body needs a certain amount and type of food to function, this will make your body slim and healthy. It's like a car. Filling it with the right fuel will work better and last longer without problems. Obesity has been shown to be one of the most common factors leading to disease and rapid aging.

Exercise also does wonders for health and psychology. It increases your metabolism and protects you from cardiovascular problems like heart attack, one of the most common ways to end someone's life in the world today.

Getting the right sleep pattern can also help. This is because the body regenerates cells faster, and a stronger immune system helps to keep you healthy from cells which can cause harmful diseases in the body.

At any cost, avoid bad habits like smoking and alcohol. They disrupt your overall health, gain weight, grow faster, destroy your immune system and cause many other problems. Instead, incorporate healthy habits into your lifestyle, such as drinking plenty of clean water every day.

CHAPTER 5
28 Days diet meal plan

A 28-Day Sample Menu for the Diet

On the diet, you will eat a Fueling or Lean & Green meal every two to three hours. (2,3,5) Below is an example of a twenty-eight-day menu for the 5&1 Plan.

DAY 1

BREAKFAST

1 cup skim or low-fat milk

¾ cup ready-to-eat unsweetened cereal

Serving Size

1 Starch

1 Dairy

Mid-Morning Fueling

Optimal Health Strawberry Yogurt Bar

Serving Size

1 Optimal Health Fueling

LUNCH

½ cup cooked cauliflower

3 oz. grilled chicken

¾ cup low-fat yogurt

Serving Size

1 Vegetable

1 Protein

1 Dairy

Mid-Afternoon Fueling

Optimal Health Strawberry Banana Smoothie

Serving

1 Optimal Health Fueling

DINNER

2 cups raw spinach

1cup total diced tomatoes, cucumbers, and mushrooms

3 oz. baked yellowfin tuna

2Tbsp low-fat salad dressing 1 small apple

Serving Size

2 Vegetables

1 Protein

1 Fat

1 Fruit

DAY 2
BREAKFAST

1 large grapefruit

3 Scrambled Eggs

Snack

25 almonds

LUNCH

Turkey Wrap

1 apple

 Snack

1 piece of string cheese

DINNER

Side salad and 2 Tbsp olive oil/vinegar dressing

Spicy Chicken and Pasta

DAY 3
BREAKFAST
1 banana

2 Tbsp of peanut butter with 1 piece of toast

Snack

2 small boxes of raisins

LUNCH
Leftover Spicy Chicken and Pasta

Snack

0% fat Greek yogurt

DINNER
2 cups of broccoli

Miso Salmon

DAY 4
BREAKFAST
1 large grapefruit

Lean Eggs and Ham

Snack

25 almonds

LUNCH
1 apple

Black Bean and Cheese Burrito

Snack

1 piece of string cheese

DINNER

1 serving of sweet potato fries

Salad with 4 Tbsp olive oil/vinegar dressing

Veggie Burger and bun

DAY 5

BREAKFAST

0% fat Greek yogurt

Berry Wafflewich

Snack

2 Tbsp of hummus

15 snap peas

LUNCH

1 apple

Gobbleguac Sandwich

Snack

1 piece of string cheese

1 banana

DINNER

2 cups of broccoli

1 cup of brown rice

Steamed Snapper with Pesto

DAY 6

BREAKFAST

1 large grapefruit

0% fat Greek yogurt

Snack

1 Luna Bar

LUNCH

25 almonds

The I-Am-Not-Eating-Salad Salad

Snack

4 Tbsp of hummus

30 baby carrots

DINNER

2 cups of snow peas

1 cup of brown rice

Chicken Spinach Parm

DAY 7

BREAKFAST

1 banana

Loaded Vegetable Omelet

Snack

1 piece of string cheese

LUNCH

1 apple

Turkey Wrap

Snack

2 Tbsp of hummus

10 cherry tomatoes

DINNER

2 cups of broccoli

Quick Lemon Chicken with Rice

Snack

1 Sugar-Free Fudgsicle

DAY 8

BREAKFAST

1 banana

Loaded Vegetable Omelet

 Snack

2 Tbsp of hummus

15 baby carrots

LUNCH

Eat Out

Snack

0% fat Greek yogurt

DINNER

2 cups of broccoli

Penne with Chicken Marengo

DAY 9

BREAKFAST

1 large grapefruit

3 Scrambled Eggs

Snack

25 almonds

 LUNCH

2 cups of broccoli

Leftover Penne with Chicken Marengo

Snack

0% fat Greek yogurt

1 piece of string cheese

DINNER

2 cups of snow peas

Thai Beef Lettuce Wraps

Snack

1 Skinny Cow ice cream sandwich

DAY 10

BREAKFAST

1 banana

Loaded Vegetable Omelet

 Snack

0% fat Greek yogurt

1 piece of string cheese

LUNCH

1 apple

The I-Am-Not-Eating-Salad Salad

Snack

1 Luna Bar

10 cherry tomatoes

DINNER

2 cups of broccoli

Tofu Stir-Fry

1 cup of brown rice

DAY 11

BREAKFAST

1 large grapefruit

3 Scrambled Eggs

 Snack

25 almonds

0% fat Greek yogurt

LUNCH

1 cup of brown rice

Leftover Tofu Stir-Fry

 Snack

1 piece of string cheese

1 banana

DINNER

2 cups of broccoli

Quick Lemon Chicken with Rice

DAY 12

BREAKFAST

1 banana

Giant Omelet Scramble

Snack

2 small boxes of raisins

LUNCH

1 apple

Turkey Wrap

Snack

1 Lärabar

DINNER

2 cups of broccoli

1 cup of brown rice

Grilled Cilantro-Lime Chicken

DAY 13

BREAKFAST

1 large grapefruit

Loaded Vegetable Omelet

Snack

1 banana

0% fat Greek yogurt

LUNCH

1 apple

Turkey Wrap

Snack

2 Tbsp of hummus

15 baby carrots

DINNER

1 cup of brown rice

2 cups of broccoli

Steamed Snapper with Pesto

DAY 14

BREAKFAST

1 medium grapefruit

Lean Eggs and Ham

Snack

25 almonds

1 piece of string cheese

LUNCH

1 apple

Mediterranean Hummus Wrap

Snack

Smart Balance Light Butter Popcorn, mini bag

DINNER

2 cups of broccoli

Penne with Chicken Marengo

Snack

30 baby carrots

DAY 15
BREAKFAST

1 large grapefruit

Don't-Get-Fat French Toast

Snack

1 piece of string cheese

2 small boxes of raisins

LUNCH

1 apple

The I-Am-Not-Eating-Salad Salad

Snack

2 Tbsp of hummus

15 baby carrots

DINNER

Salad with 2 Tbsp olive oil/vinegar dressing

Miso Salmon

DAY 16

BREAKFAST

1 large grapefruit

Loaded Vegetable Omelet

Snack

Smart Balance Light Butter Popcorn, mini bag

LUNCH

1 apple

Mediterranean Hummus Wrap

Snack

0% fat Greek yogurt

DINNER

2 cups of broccoli

Whole Wheat Pasta with Vegetables

Snack

1 Skinny Cow ice cream sandwich

DAY 17

BREAKFAST

1 large grapefruit

Giant Omelet Scramble

Snack

1 piece of string cheese

LUNCH

1 apple

Leftover Whole Wheat Pasta with Vegetables

Snack

25 almonds

DINNER

1 cup of brown rice

Tofu Stir-Fry

DAY 18

BREAKFAST

1 large grapefruit

Belly-Stuffing Peanut Butter Oatmeal

Snack

1 piece of string cheese

LUNCH

1 cup of brown rice

Leftover Tofu Stir-Fry

Snack

0% fat Greek yogurt

DINNER

Salad with 2 Tbsp olive oil/vinegar dressing

2 cups of broccoli

Chicken Spinach Parm

DAY 19

BREAKFAST

1 large grapefruit

Lean Eggs and Ham

Snack

1 banana

0% fat Greek yogurt

LUNCH

Gobbleguac Sandwich

Snack

1 piece of string cheese

DINNER

2 cups of broccoli

1 cup of brown rice

Steamed Snapper with Pesto

DAY 20

BREAKFAST

Don't-Get-Fat French Toast

Snack

2 small boxes of raisins

1 banana

LUNCH

1 apple

The I-Am-Not-Eating-Salad Salad

Snack

1 piece of string cheese

2 Tbsp of hummus

15 baby carrots

DINNER

Salad with 2 Tbsp olive oil/vinegar dressing

Miso Salmon

DAY 21

BREAKFAST

1 large grapefruit

2 Tbsp of peanut butter with 1 piece of whole-grain toast

Snack

25 almonds

LUNCH

1 apple

Gobbleguac Sandwich

Snack

1 piece of string cheese

DINNER

Eat Out

DAY 22

BREAKFAST

1 banana

Loaded Vegetable Omelet

Snack

1 Luna Bar

LUNCH

1 apple

Black Bean and Cheese Burrito

Snack

2 small boxes of raisins

DINNER

Salad with 2 Tbsp olive oil/vinegar dressing

Grilled Cilantro-Lime Chicken

Snack

1 sugar-free Fudgsicle

DAY 23

BREAKFAST

1 banana

Loaded Vegetable Omelet

Snack

1 Luna Bar

LUNCH

1 apple

Black Bean and Cheese Burrito

Snack

2 small boxes of raisins

DINNER

Salad with 2 Tbsp olive oil/vinegar dressing

Whole Wheat Pasta with Vegetables

Snack

1 Skinny Cow ice cream sandwich

DAY 24
BREAKFAST
1 large grapefruit

Giant Omelet Scramble

Snack

1 piece of string cheese

LUNCH
1 apple

Leftover Whole Wheat Pasta with Vegetables

Snack

25 almonds

DINNER
1 cup of brown rice

Miso Salmon

DAY 25
BREAKFAST
1 large grapefruit

Berry Wafflewich

Snack

30 baby carrots

0% fat Greek yogurt

LUNCH
1 apple

Gobbleguac Sandwich

Snack

1 piece of string cheese

DINNER

1/2 cup of brown rice

2 cups of broccoli

Tofu Stir-fry

Snack

1 Skinny Cow ice cream sandwich

DAY 26

BREAKFAST

1 large grapefruit

Belly-Stuffing Peanut Butter Oatmeal

Snack

0% fat Greek yogurt

LUNCH

2 cups of broccoli

Leftover Tofu Stir-fry

Snack

30 baby carrots

25 almonds

DINNER

1/2 cup of brown rice

Chicken Spinach Parm

Snack

1 Skinny Cow ice cream sandwich

DAY 27
BREAKFAST
0% fat Greek yogurt

Giant Omelet Scramble

Snack

1 Luna Bar

LUNCH
1 apple

Black Bean and Cheese Burrito

DINNER
1 serving of sweet potato fries

Salad with 2 Tbsp olive oil/vinegar dressing

Veggie Burger and bun

Snack

1 piece of string cheese

DAY 28
BREAKFAST
1 large grapefruit

2 Tbsp of peanut butter with 1 piece of whole-grain toast

Snack

2 Tbsp of hummus

10 cherry tomatoes

LUNCH
Mediterranean Hummus Wrap

Snack

25 almonds

0% fat Greek yogurt

DINNER

Eat Out

CPSIA information can be obtained
at www.ICGtesting.com
Printed in the USA
LVHW011307010621
689027LV00007B/575